UNPROCESSED

How the Food We Eat Is Fuelling Our Mental Health Crisis

Kimberley Wilson

WH
ALLEN

1

WH Allen, an imprint of Ebury Publishing
20 Vauxhall Bridge Road
London SW1V 2SA

WH Allen is part of the Penguin Random House group of companies
whose addresses can be found at global.penguinrandomhouse.com

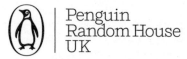

First published by WH Allen in 2023

www.penguin.co.uk

A CIP catalogue record for this book is available from the British Library

ISBN 9780753559741

Typeset in 10.5/15.5pt ITC Galliard Pro by Jouve (UK), Milton Keynes
Printed and bound in Great Britain by Clays Ltd, Elcograf S.p.A.

The authorised representative in the EEA by Penguin Random House Ireland,
Morrison Chambers, 32 Nassau Street, Dublin D02 YH68

Penguin Random House is committed to a sustainable future
for our business, our readers and our planet. This book is made
from Forest Stewardship Council® certified paper.

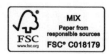

To every child who ever wonders whether anybody cares. We do.

CONTENTS

PREFACE

IN THIS BOOK I will outline the evidence on the role of nutrition on brain development, function and mental health across the human lifespan, from preconception to old age. In doing so I don't claim that nutrition is a panacea, rather a central yet overlooked and ignored underlying factor in our rising rates of mental illness and what I perceive as increased neurological vulnerability.

I have adopted the use of the term 'brain-body' to highlight the fundamentally inseparable nature of the relationship between the two. When speaking of one or the other I will say either 'brain' or 'body', but please hold in mind that any distinction is more linguistic than truly meaningful.

I was deeply honoured and proud to learn in 2022 that my first book, *How to Build a Healthy Brain*, was endorsed by the NHS as a trusted source of health information, one of only ten books to be recognised in this way. As a result, the book has been made available to every NHS England library and all UK prison libraries.

My ambition with *Unprocessed* is to maintain those high standards. As such, where I describe the effects of a particular nutrient on a health outcome, I have done my best to report naturalistically relevant doses. That is, doses that are achievable from normal (if healthy) dietary consumption or supplementation that is economically and practically feasible, and safe, for most people. Furthermore, the evidence presented is predominantly drawn from randomised controlled trials on human participants, or meta-analyses. Where results being described were conducted with animal test subjects, I have made this clear. This book has also been independently fact-checked. As a reader the downside to this careful approach is that animal data often produces more sensational results, the kind that make a splash on newspaper front pages. However, these results are too often completely irrelevant to humans. My aim is to present you with data that is accurate, informative, practical and relevant to you. That said, much of the evidence I present is *truly fascinating* and groundbreaking. It should make you feel informed and empowered but also, perhaps, a little angry. That is certainly how I feel knowing that in many cases my government has sat on research (sometimes for decades) showing that better nutrition can improve attention and memory in children, reduce our vulnerability to depression, and even lower rates of violence. Instead of acting resolutely to improve population nutrition our ministers argue among themselves, using public health policy as a bargaining chip to maintain their own positions.

Though this is very disheartening I am not quite ready to sit quietly and let this go on unchallenged. I want to at least feel that I did something. I hope you feel the same way. If you do, please join me in taking action. Throughout this book you will find information and opportunities to **Take Action** and make your voice heard, whether that is through sharing something on social media or writing to your MP. You don't have to care about every single subject I raise in this book. Perhaps you have a particular interest in maternal nutrition. Or maybe your life has been touched by dementia and that is where you want to focus your energy. What matters is that you participate. Speak up. Be heard.

What's on the Menu?

For those of you who like to plan your consumption in advance here is what you can expect. The book is laid out in broadly chronological order. I start in **Part I** by considering the history of mental illness and outlining the evolutionary justification for the essential role of certain nutrients for human brain and mental health. In the remainder of the book I look at the evidence of the impact of our modern diets on brain health from preconception to older age.

Lifelong mental wellness has its foundations in pregnancy and this is the focus of **Part II**. **The Maternal Universe** and **The Importance of DHA** chapters may be of particular interest to anyone in a position to advise pregnant women and families (e.g. GPs, midwives, obstetricians, gynaecologists, fertility professionals), childcare professionals and educators, as well as the parents of young children or parents-to-be.

If you want to skip the starters and really get your teeth stuck into the effects our modern diets are having on our brains and society head straight to **Parts III** and **IV**, where we kick off with **Sugar** and **Ultra-Processed Foods** and cover everything from **Alcohol** to **Veganism**.

You can think of **Part V** as the after-dinner espresso; a little pick-me-up to see you on your way. Here, I look at the current barriers to implementing important public health policy that could improve the nutrient status and mental health outcomes of the population, as well as offering some practical solutions.

As a self-confessed nerd and feeder I provide you with a substantial serving of the freshest science as well as some food for thought. I hope at the end of this book you will feel full of new knowledge but also energised. May what you read here sustain any positive actions you take for yourself, your loved ones, your community.

Who Should Foot the Bill?

One day a butler knocks on your door. When you open it, he explains that you have been selected to make the showstopper dessert for a VIP state dinner. You're whizzed off to a brightly lit, modern kitchen stocked with every ingredient imaginable. Shelves of flour of every conceivable grain. Dozens of sugars, syrups and honeys. Fruit, chocolate, nuts, sprinkles and glazes. You have everything you need and you can pick anything you like. You look down at the recipe you have been given:

Select ingredients.
Make dish.

Despite your best efforts, care and enthusiasm, the odds of success are not stacked in your favour. Because it doesn't matter how much 'choice' you have if you don't have sufficient information and guidance. Nutrition matters for brain development and mental health but not all the foods we encounter in our modern food environments are up to the job. But how are you supposed to know that?

Please bear this in mind as you read this book. My intention is not to point fingers or blame parents for not eating 'correctly' during pregnancy or not feeding their children 'the right things'. Rather, my argument is that we (parents and the public) have inadequate, insufficient and out-of-date information on the impact of nutrition on brain health, and unequal access to nutritious foods. The government has an obligation to make important health information available and accessible so that people may then act on it. It has a responsibility to enact health policy to support the physical and mental health of the population. In these duties of care, it is my case that the government is failing.

STRONGER FOUNDATIONS

THE JAPANESE ARCHIPELAGO sits on one of the most seismically active regions in the world. The islands are located on the dramatically titled 'Pacific Ring of Fire' where several tectonic plates meet, the resulting geological friction making the region prone to volcanic eruptions, frequent earthquakes and catastrophic tsunamis. Japan typically experiences thousands of small quakes and at least one moderate to strong earthquake (one that results in property damage or loss of life) every year.

For the Japanese, earthquakes are, to an extent, a part of life. This is captured in some of the nation's proverbs. *Jishin kaminari kaji oyaji* lists the things most feared by the Japanese: 'earthquakes, thunderbolts, fires, fathers' (assuming this list is ranked in ascending order, the patriarchs of feudal Japan were evidently quite the force to be reckoned with). Then there is the more encouraging *Nanakorobi yaoki*: 'Fall seven times, stand up eight'. I find it fitting that this invitation to rise again after a fall should emerge from a nation that has been forced to rebuild several times following devastating earthquakes and the associated tsunamis. It is a quintessential message of resilience in the face of a high degree of terrestrial disquiet, an ongoing risk that they have to find a way to live with.

To mitigate this persistent risk, earthquake-resistant building regulations were introduced in Japan in 1924. These policies were a response to the deadly magnitude 7.9 earthquake that struck the Kantō

Plain in September 1923. An estimated 142,000 people were killed, with millions left homeless.

A series of new regulations put in place in the 1920s required buildings to be constructed with reinforced concrete and set a minimum thickness for wooden beams in town housing. Buildings built to these regulations are referred to as *kyu-taishin*, where *kyu* (旧) means 'prior' and *taishin* (耐震) means 'resistance'. When, in 1978, an earthquake in the Miyagi prefecture killed 28 people, completely destroyed over 800 homes and damaged thousands more, these policies were tightened further, and from then on all new buildings were to be constructed to withstand magnitude 7 quakes.

Crucially, these successive interventions worked. Today, state-of-the-art Japanese buildings are constructed with 'base isolation': the building is designed to float on specially designed shock-absorbing foundations, protecting the structure from direct contact with the earth and reducing the amount of vibration that reverberates up into the building that can cause damage. There are even eyewitness reports that in a base-isolated building during the magnitude 6.9 'Great Hanshin' quake of 1995, movement was so dampened that books stayed on the shelves.

The Power of Policy

This superior earthquake resistance, and the many precious lives it has saved, is really an elegant example of the power of policy. In response to an identifiable but uncontrollable environmental risk the Japanese set about strengthening and fortifying their buildings to be more resilient to those risks, from the foundations up. They identified the vulnerabilities and sought to control the controllables.

Here is what the Japanese did not do. They did not simply invest in superficially repairing the damaged buildings in the hope that they would function 'well enough' until the next quake. A hasty paint job and some filler to hide the cracks would have made some buildings presentable but no less fragile. They also did not just continue to build their buildings to the same inadequate standards. To do so would have been an act of gross negligence, a disaster waiting to happen.

Yet, to my mind, the 'superficial repair' strategy is analogous to the UK's overarching approach to a very different, but potentially even more harmful threat: population mental health. We wait for the earthquake to strike and then try to do a bit of a patch-up job. We do enough, perhaps, to get the person back to work – with the cracks showing but still, to quote the earthquake regulations, 'continuing to function as normal' (or at least appearing to) – and then cross our fingers and hope that another 'earthquake' doesn't hit.

We do not invest in reinforcing the foundations of mental health: building resilient brains.

Here's the problem, though: the earthquake has already hit. Common mental health concerns (depression and anxiety), neurodevelopmental disorders such as ADHD (attention deficit hyperactivity disorder), and rates of self-harm in young people have been increasing in the UK for decades, largely driven by worsening mental health in 18- to 25-year-olds. While some of this increased incidence may be down to better diagnosis, hard data points like A&E attendance and self-harm rates indicate that our mental health and psychological resilience are objectively worsening. These are the signs that our brains are like pre-regulation buildings in Japan; they are vulnerable. And this vulnerability is evident when we look at the mental health statistics.

More people than ever are becoming ill:

- Mental illness is the second leading cause of disease burden in England and rates have been steadily rising for 30 years.
- The rates of probable mental disorder in children aged 5–16 have risen from one in nine in 2017 to one in six in 2020.
- 27.2 per cent of young women and 13.3 per cent of young men (aged 17–22) have a probable mental health disorder.

There isn't enough treatment:

- Only around a quarter of people with common mental health conditions receive treatment.

- Yet, the median time for a young person to access therapy in the UK is 60 days, with some waiting up to 345 days. The majority of adults have to wait over six months. (I know of a two-year waiting list for specialist ADHD treatment.)
- GPs describe being forced to prescribe antidepressants because psychological therapy is unavailable in their area.

The treatments we do have are failing:

- Only around half of people referred to talking therapy treatment recover.
- Up to 30 per cent of those diagnosed with depression in the UK have treatment-resistant depression, a total of 2.7 million people.

So, we have a mental health landscape in which more people, including children and adolescents, are becoming ill, too few receive treatment, and those who do often have to wait several months for it, during which time their mental health is likely to further deteriorate, making the illness more intractable and harder to treat. And for those with the most common mental health problems only about half will recover. What happens to the 76 per cent who don't receive treatment in the first place?

The Covid-19 pandemic constitutes another major mental health earthquake. Early data from the Care Quality Commission, the independent regulator for health and social care in England, shows that there was a near 5 per cent increase in the number of people being detained under the Mental Health Act. The increase is attributed to the negative impact of reduced access to mental health services during the pandemic. Those whose mental health was more vulnerable before the pandemic were hardest hit, with twice the proportion of single parents, the unemployed and those with long-term health conditions reporting suicidal thoughts compared to the overall population, and households in receipt of benefits experiencing higher rates of distress.

The mental health charity Mind reports that 65 per cent of adults and 68 per cent of young people stated that their mental health had worsened since the first national lockdown. However, the major aftershocks – the long-term impact on the nation of two years of uncontrollable stress – remain to be felt.

If we think things are bad now (and most people on the front line of mental health provision do) then the future looks catastrophic. A rise in the number of children with neuropsychiatric disorders means more of our young people will experience poorer quality of life and more mental health difficulties, as well as placing greater demand on parents and additional stress on the quality of family life. In terms of the wider social impact, attending to the needs of children with neuropsychiatric disorders has been found to reduce parents' productivity, earning potential and contribution to the economy, as well as being associated with higher use of health services. In adults, mental health conditions are already one of the leading causes of sickness absence in the UK and they are the primary cause of sick days for NHS staff. Finally, outside of Covid, dementia and Alzheimer's disease are the leading cause of death in the UK. With global cases of dementia set to triple in the next 30 years, we are facing a looming care crisis that could cripple both the health service and the economy. We literally *can't afford* for things to get worse.

Something is disastrously wrong with the way that we understand and treat mental illness. Our buildings are crumbling and yet we just keep painting over the cracks with conversations that don't seem to actually change anything. It won't be long before the tide of un- and under-treated mental illness in the UK becomes a tidal wave that overwhelms our already stretched health service and triggers more 'deaths of despair' – the increased alcohol, drug and suicide mortality in those who feel their lives are no longer worth living.

What we urgently need is an overhaul in our understanding of mental health with a focus on prevention, risk reduction, early intervention and resilience. Though we can't control external factors like pandemics or earthquakes, we can, the evidence suggests, reinforce and fortify our brain architecture. This means planning ahead for the brains we want to build, rather than leaving it to chance. It means learning from experience. Just like the Japanese contractors, we must go right back to the foundations.

Building Blocks

An architect or builder selects the right materials for the job. Some bricks are porous, others heat-resistant, others contain higher levels of minerals, some can resist acid. Ultimately, the quality of the bricks will influence the overall quality, durability and resilience of the structure. It is the same for your brain.

You will have heard much about the mental health crisis, about the negative effects of social media and the need to reduce stigma. These things matter but there is a greater untold story about the origins of our troubles. While there are many pieces to the puzzle of mental health it makes sense to focus on the structure from which mental health emerges. The literal building blocks of the brain are nutrients. The evolution of our exquisite brains depended on the availability of key materials, and you need an adequate supply of the right nutritional 'bricks' to build a resilient brain. When this doesn't happen, the result is poorer brain development and increased vulnerability to mental illness.

In this book you will learn that:

- If a mother doesn't eat enough of the right fats during pregnancy her baby's brain is smaller and less well connected. She is also more likely to give birth prematurely, which brings its own brain-development risks for baby. Most women don't know this.
- There is a nutrient that, when supplemented during pregnancy, has been shown to prevent the brain changes associated with autism and schizophrenia. It also increases children's attention years later (a major predictor of children's school achievement). Most health professionals don't know this.
- Just a few days on a diet of high-sugar, high-fat, ultra-processed foods leads to measurable impairment in learning, memory and

appetite control. Long-term diets high in these foods are linked to increased risk and severity of depression, especially in young people. Most politicians, who are responsible for the policies around the marketing of these foods, don't seem to care about this.

Every day you make several decisions – consciously or unconsciously – about what to eat, how to prepare it, and how much of it to consume. The nutrients you ingest influence the structure of your brain, the production of brain chemicals that create your mood, and the speed at which your brain ages. Yet if you go to your doctor for help with a mental health issue, you're more likely to be asked about your relationship with your mother than what you had for breakfast. Hardly anyone, especially those in positions of power and influence, is paying attention to the clear link between what we eat, how we feel, and who we are. I want them, and you, to come away from this book understanding how the foods a pregnant woman eats influence her baby's IQ, why we're eating our way to Alzheimer's and whether nutrient deficiencies can make you violent. There will be novel insights but not all of this information is new. Some researchers have been ringing the early warning alarm bell on food and the brain for 50 years. It's time we started listening.

Ultimately, I want to help you to understand how our changing food environment and eating habits are contributing to the rise in psychological distress so that you can either make changes for yourself or demand more and better from your policymakers. Importantly, unlike earthquakes, the food environment isn't uncontrollable. We can make it better if we really want to. Let's not sit idly by, waiting for the tsunami to hit. With the evidence presented in this book, the results of thousands of clinical studies over the decades, we have the opportunity to turn the tide, to start to build stronger and more resilient brains from the moment of conception, if not before.

We're going to start, though, with a whistle-stop tour through mental illness: what we've historically got wrong about it, and what we continue to get wrong today.

PART I

OUR ANCIENT ARCHITECTURE

CHAPTER 1

A BRIEF HISTORY OF MENTAL ILLNESS – FROM MYSTICS AND MAGIC . . . TO THE MUNDANE

SINCE YOU HAVE picked up this book, I'll assume that you have an interest in how food affects the brain. However, you (for the moment at least) are in something of a minority. When we think about the things that increase someone's risk of, say, depression we typically consider their past experiences, their current relationships, their future hopes. We tend not to consider their nutrition. And that's not just the general public. Many GPs, psychologists and psychiatrists, including many in powerful positions in their respective fields, are resistant to the idea that current or past nutrition has something to do with why our patients feel so bad. So why do we find it so hard to think about food in this way? Because it goes against hundreds of years of mental health tradition that, broadly, considered the mind to be separate from the body.

Before the modern era of neuroscience and psychology, mental illness was understood to be evidence of the supernatural: a sign of demonic possession, unhappy deities or vengeful curses. As far back as

6500BC it was common to drill holes in the skull to aid the release of the evil spirits that had become trapped there and were believed to be responsible for the symptoms of mental illness, a practice called trephination. These supernatural beliefs were widespread, with evidence of trephination uncovered in ancient burial sites in Peru, France, Kenya and China, and such beliefs are well documented in both the Old and New Testaments. The book of Deuteronomy, for example, describes mental illness as a punishment from God, with the Israelites warned that 'The Lord shall smite thee with madness' should they misbehave.

At various points, early modern thinkers dabbled with the idea that there may instead be a physical basis, rather than a supernatural one, for mental health problems. For the ancient Egyptians, Mesopotamians and ancient Greeks mental illness in women was evidence of a 'wandering uterus': the term 'hysteria' takes its name from the ancient Greek *hustérā*, meaning 'womb'. The Greek physician, Hippocrates (c. 460≈377BC) wrote that 'if a woman's uterus moves against her liver, she will suddenly lose her speech, grind her teeth, and take on a livid colouring'. Treatments for this itinerant organ involved using scents to guide the uterus back to its rightful position. The term 'hysteria' was later borrowed into early psychoanalysis, which ascribed neurosis, particularly in women, to repressed memories or sexual urges. And it was the same Hippocrates who came up with the idea of the 'four humours' to explain mental illness, whereby symptoms were attributed to an imbalance of bodily fluids. In this tradition, for example, an excess of black bile was believed to make someone melancholic. The 'cure' was to rebalance the fluids through such (perilous and ineffective) treatments as purging and bloodletting.

However, the movement towards more natural causes for psychological distress did not last long. The Middle Ages saw the return of the supernatural as the origin of mental ill health; that is to say, as the Church regained power so did the demons. Afflictions like the Black Death were variously interpreted as acts of the devil, punishments from God, or witchcraft.

The Mind-Body Problem – and the Problem with Descartes

The backdrop to this centuries-old battle between angry gods and imbalanced bodies is the search for a satisfactory resolution to the mind-body problem. On the one hand we have a body, which, though impressive, is not too different (and in many ways inferior to) the bodies of other animals. Yet, we possess a mind that is capable of seemingly unique human faculties – imagination, emotion, language and so on. How does a run-of-the-mill physical body (or brain) give rise to such wondrous complexity? Our thoughts, dreams, ambitions *feel* like they arise independently of our bodies. How can they possibly be connected? Four centuries ago, one man offered a solution to this problem, the ripples of which are still felt today: René Descartes.

Cartesian dualism is the proposition that humans have two distinct and separable properties: physical and mental, matter and mind. Not only that, but that the mind (not the brain) is the thing solely responsible for conscious thought – the body plays no role in thinking. In later chapters I will present modern neuroscience evidence that emphatically proves this to be wrong. Nonetheless, the theory of a mind that is separate from its body has influenced policies on issues as diverse as legal culpability for murder and the best treatment for depression in the 400 years since it was proposed and widely adopted.

Fast-forward to 2023 and the modern-day bibles of mental health, the US-based *Diagnostic and Statistical Manual of Mental Disorders* (DSM) and the World Health Organization's International Classification of Diseases (ICD). These are classification systems for psychiatric illnesses. They are put together by panels of experts, revised every decade or so and provide healthcare professionals with the symptom criteria for an illness diagnosis. For example, in order to be diagnosed with depression the most recent revision of the DSM, version 5, dictates that a person must be experiencing five or more of the symptoms listed on the following page during the same two-week period, and at least one of the symptoms should be either (1) depressed mood or (2) loss of interest or pleasure.

1. Depressed mood most of the day, nearly every day.
2. Markedly diminished interest or pleasure in all, or almost all, activities most of the day, nearly every day.
3. Significant weight loss when not dieting or weight gain, or decrease or increase in appetite nearly every day.
4. A slowing down of thought and a reduction of physical movement (observable by others, not merely subjective feelings of restlessness or being slowed down).
5. Fatigue or loss of energy nearly every day.
6. Feelings of worthlessness or excessive or inappropriate guilt nearly every day.
7. Diminished ability to think or concentrate, or indecisiveness, nearly every day.
8. Recurrent thoughts of death, recurrent suicidal ideation without a specific plan, or a suicide attempt or a specific plan for committing suicide.

To receive a diagnosis of depression, these symptoms must cause significant distress or impairment in work or life functioning, and must not be caused by substance abuse or another medical condition.

With each subsequent revision the number of diagnostic categories increases, from 102 when it was published in 1952, to around 300 in the 2013 edition. Some of these changes reflect better understanding or a greater specificity in the classification of illnesses.

However, despite the plethora of diagnostic categories, there is little consensus on the *causes* of depression (or other mental illness). The dominant hypothesis for depression, for example (see box on next page), has always been unable to explain *why* brain chemistry apparently becomes unbalanced, and has now been abandoned by most researchers. So, doctors will now be able to tell you with some degree of confidence that you *are* depressed, but not what that means about what is happening in your brain-body. Your thinking is off and you feel bad but we don't know *why*. This is why I believe that for all our progress, in a way we still have gods in the mental health consulting room: because we still commonly think about the mind as separate from the body.

THE SEROTONIN HYPOTHESIS

Serotonin is a neuronal-signalling molecule, which plays a role in a wide range of processes including mood regulation, learning, memory and gut motility.

The serotonin hypothesis of depression proposes that depression is caused by insufficient production or uptake of serotonin in the brain. Selective serotonin reuptake inhibitors are a class of antidepressant medication designed to relieve depression by increasing serotonin availability and activity in the brain.

However, while these types of drugs do work for some people with (especially severe) depression, their efficacy for mild to moderate depression is lower than would be hoped or predicted from the proposed mechanism of action.

Serotonin is likely to play a regulatory or modulatory role in mood function; however, the evidence indicates that the hypothesis that depression is the result of an insufficiency of serotonin is overly simplistic and inaccurate.

We talk about psychological trauma and pain as afflictions of the mind and not the brain-body. The psychiatric separation of the mind and body should be thought of as the final vestige of thousands of years of supernatural explanations for mental illness. The serotonin hypothesis feels to me to be a modern rendering of Hippocrates' four humours.

In over 20 years of psychology training and practice I received little formal instruction on the physiological (rather than the sociocultural) relationship between my patients' bodies and their brains. In lectures we (rightly) discussed the impact of being abused; poor; female; of an ethnic minority; or at risk for things like depression and psychosis; but nothing on the impact of being malnourished or hungry on brain development, mood and mental wellbeing. The body, we came to understand, was only relevant in what it *symbolised* in the social world;

it only mattered as far as what it made other people think about you, influenced how they treated you, or what it caused you to think about yourself. What was *happening* in the body and how that linked to mood or any other psychological symptom didn't get a mention. Similarly, medical trainings rarely cover the role of nutrition on psychiatric presentations except perhaps in the case of vitamin B12 deficiency, which is known to cause depression, irritability and problems with memory and judgement. This, of course, begs the question: why would we suppose that only this one deficiency among all the nutrients essential for life would impact us in this way?

So, overwhelmingly, mental health disorders are treated as 'mind' problems that have nothing to do with the conditions within, or contributions of, the body. A patient who presents with depression is more likely to be asked about their relationship with their mother than their relationship with food or exercise.

Putting the Mind Back in the Body

We still think of the mind as mystical because we don't yet have sufficiently advanced technology to understand it. Encased in the thick shell of the skull its actions are not readily observable, which means that even key functions like the glymphatic system are still only just being discovered.

Yet, we are making good progress with technologies and methodologies for understanding the brain. We know, for example, what brain cells are made of. We know that the building blocks of the brain are certain nutrients that must come directly from the diet. We know that there are crucial periods during brain development in utero and infancy when these nutrients are more important. While there is still much to be understood about the role of neurotransmitters such as serotonin and their involvement in brain function, we know that in order to synthesise these chemicals certain nutrients need to be in adequate supply. We know that nutritional status influences stress resilience. And we know, for sure, that fewer and fewer of us are getting enough of these building blocks of a healthy brain.

Scientific progress is characterised by the transition from the super-natural to the natural, from the mystical to the mundane. For thousands of years we thought the gods controlled the weather. But now it's just physics. This is the transition we are currently in with mental health; moving from a mind that is mysterious and 'out there' to one that is an indelible product of a physical brain in a physical body. But change is hard. When you have learned, taught and prescribed one way of thinking about mental health, shifting those established beliefs is difficult. It might mean assimilating a whole new research field or (which is even harder) abandoning some long-held 'truths'. It might occasion a trans-formation in personal or professional identity. While these kinds of paradigm shifts can be thrilling, they can also be unsettling and hard to swallow. For Descartes the mind was proof of the existence of God. But that was 400 years ago. And while I am not suggesting that nutri-tion answers all of our questions around the mind and mental health, it is a key and undervalued part of the overall picture. A better under-standing and acceptance of the role of food and nutrition in building healthy, resilient brains, and in treatment and recovery, enables us to make better decisions for ourselves, our patients and our citizens.

Throughout this book I will use the stories of two ordinary women and their children to illustrate the profound influence of habitual diet on the brain and mental health across the average lifespan. There is, quite deliberately, nothing special about these characters: where pos-sible I have based their milestones on UK population averages.

CHAPTER 2

REIGN OF THE FAT HEADS

COMPARED TO OTHER animals the human body is – how can I put this kindly? – not very impressive. We're not as fast as cheetahs. We can't fly. We're nowhere near as strong as our chimp cousins. But there is something else that allowed us to forge ahead as a species: the ability to think. More specifically, the capacity for self-awareness, to imagine, plan, test, learn and communicate through written and spoken language and the plethora of other cognitive capabilities that distinguish us from even our closest primate relatives. What is it about the human brain that makes us stand out from the crowd?

One thing is size. Humans have the biggest brains relative to body size of the large land mammals. The brain of an African elephant, the largest land mammal, is 0.1 per cent of its total body mass. Our closest primate relative, the chimpanzee, has a brain that is 0.8 per cent of its overall body weight. *Homo sapiens* weigh in with a brain that is 2 per cent of our body weight. I know on the face of it that doesn't sound like very much, but you'll soon see why this is so extraordinary.

There is another, more sophisticated measure of an animal's brain size. Encephalisation quotient (EQ) is the ratio of the actual size of an animal's brain compared to what you would predict the volume to be based on that animal's size and shape. Here again humans outstrip other species.

Comparing Differences in Encephalisation Quotient (EQ) between Humans and Other Animals

Species	Encephalisation quotient (EQ)
Human	7.4–7.8
Bottlenose dolphin	4.14
Chimpanzee	2.2–2.5
Rhesus monkey	2.1
African elephant	1.13
Dog	1.2
Cat	1.0
Horse	0.9
Sheep	0.8
Mouse	0.5
Rat	0.4
Rabbit	0.4
Whale	0.18

So, a cat's brain is roughly the size you would expect for its size and body shape, a whale's much smaller, and a human's much bigger. For other land-based mammals brain size reduces logarithmically in relation to body size. But not us. We are the heavyweights of the brain world. This additional capacity seems to give us an advantage when it comes to navigating complex societies and diverse cultures. And though size isn't everything, this unusually large endowment is worth remarking on because the size of an animal's brain is limited by two major factors: energy and nutrient availability.

Brains are very, very expensive to run in terms of energy. Though it accounts for just 2 per cent of body weight the human brain has a huge energy requirement and is responsible for about 23 per cent of adult basal metabolic rate, the number of calories you burn when your body is at rest. For a baby, whose brain comprises a larger proportion of its overall body mass, that figure rises to 74 per cent. That means that the biggest single contribution to your body's metabolic rate is your brain.

But, as we all know, bills have to be paid: the larger the brain, the higher the energy requirement – in other words, the more fuel the animal needs to consume on a daily basis. Evolution manages this dilemma in a number of ways. One is to limit the size of the body relative to the brain. Another is to give us a preference for energy-dense foods (more on this later). Yet another is to eat a lot. Our closest evolutionary cousins, chimpanzees, have very little body fat (the body's energy storage facility) and spend 6–8 hours per day eating to provide their bodies and brains with sufficient energy (see table below). And while this sounds like the height of luxury (or me on holiday), spending most of your day eating in order to survive is a huge limitation on freedom and the ability to do other things. In fact, some researchers believe that it is, at least in part, the genetic mutation that allows humans to store fat that has contributed to the evolution of our big brains and complex social lives. When you can store fat, you can, effectively, take your energy with you. This allows the individual (and the group) to be more mobile, freeing them up to travel to new landscapes and habitats. It also liberates your hands: rather than being occupied picking fruit, digging tubers and holding on to branches, our hands were free to fashion tools, build fire, sculpt pots, all of which contributed to the evolution of our culture.

Energy Consumption Differences between Bonobo Chimpanzees and Humans

	Bonobo chimpanzees	Humans
Male body fat %	0.005	5.2–30.2
Female body fat %	3.6	9.4–54.1
Skin as % of total body weight	10–13*	5.6–6.1
Hours per day spent feeding	6–8	2–3**

* To compensate for having less body fat, chimps have thicker skin than humans, which helps them to retain body heat.
** For the size of our brains it's estimated that we *should* have to eat for 9+ hours per day.

Finally, having extra time provides the opportunity to *think*. If you are not constantly scanning the ground for something to eat you can turn your head to the horizon and track the angle of the sun, or look up at the night sky and begin to wonder what those spots of light might be. Fat storage gifted us thinking time.

The other distinguishing feature of the human brain is the size and connectivity of the prefrontal cortex (PFC), the part of the brain that allows us to weigh up options, predict outcomes, make decisions and behave in a deliberate manner. Humans have a proportionally larger PFC compared to other higher primates and this is understood to account for much of our capacity for more complex cognition and language.

So, our brains are large, well connected and come with a generous PFC. We can store fat, which helps us to be able to afford these expensive, fuel-guzzling organs. But that doesn't explain why we, of all the land mammals, have such outsized brains. There's more to it. Our brain is not just a static machine that only needs energy to run, like a car. It's more like a house: it requires a range of different materials to build it (concrete foundations, brick walls, glass windows) and these materials will need to be regularly maintained, updated and replaced. Holes have to be patched and extensions built. These materials, the fabric of your brain, are nutrients. And one nutrient in particular seems to hold the key to our big brains: fat.

Omega-3s

Fats are typically composed of a strip of a compound called glycerol with three fatty acid chains hanging from it. Fatty acids are composed of combinations of carbon, hydrogen and oxygen chemical elements. Fats are described as having differing levels of saturation. If you imagine the fatty acid molecule as a long dining table, the kind you see in depictions of medieval banquets, you can visualise the level of saturation as the number of people (hydrogens) sitting at the table compared to the number of empty chairs. In a saturated fat, such as those found in butter, all of the seats at the table are taken and everyone stays in their chair. This makes these fats very stable, and their orderly configuration is why these saturated fats are solid at room temperature.

Then there are the unsaturated fats (like those in olive oil), dining tables that have a bend in their formation and where not every seat is full. This means that these fats do not stack so neatly but flow and move around one another. This movement creates fluidity in the fat's structure and these fats tend to be liquid at room temperature.

The omega-3 fats are considered very long-chain highly unsaturated/polyunsaturated fatty acids. These are very long tables where there are many available seats, creating lots of flexibility in the structure of the fat. Though there are many types of omega-3, the ones we know to be essential to human health are:

- Alpha-linolenic acid (ALA)
- Eicosapentaenoic acid (EPA)
- Docosahexaenoic acid (DHA)

You are likely to have heard something about this interesting family of fats in the news or seen them on the supplement shelves. It has been shown that supplementation with them can lower the risk of heart disease and heart attacks by reducing the levels of other fat circulating in the bloodstream and reducing the 'stickiness' of blood. While it is true that what is good for the heart is good for the brain, this is not the reason that I want to talk about them. I want to tell you about their direct role in the architecture of your brain.

Although omega-3s are incorporated into the membranes of every cell in your body, they are particularly enriched in the retina, heart muscle and brain. And the fact that these distinct fats are found in such high concentrations in these tissues suggests that they play a special function in their activity. The brain is one of the fattiest organs in the body, second only to fat tissue itself. Some 60 per cent of the dry weight of the brain is fat – so, if you were to take a human brain and leave it in the sun to dry out completely over half of what would be left would be fats, and 20–25 per cent of that would be DHA, that third item on the list above, alone. What is it doing? Just to give you a sense of why there's so much DHA concentrated in your brain, let's take a very quick look at just some of its functions.

Neurogenesis

The formation of a new brain cell (neurogenesis) takes place in three stages:

1. **Proliferation** – Neural stem cells divide and begin to change shape, becoming neural precursors.
2. **Migration** – New neurones move from their location of 'birth' to their ultimate destination.
3. **Differentiation** – Newborn precursors differentiate into distinct types of brain cell and start to form neuronal circuits.

Neurogenesis takes place both in the developing brain during pregnancy and in some regions of the adult brain, and DHA is required for *each* stage.

Cell signalling

Neuronal cells communicate through chemical signals triggered by an electrical impulse (action potential). Microscopic sacs called vesicles filled with molecules of neurotransmitters (such as serotonin or dopamine) sit at the ends of the axon terminal. When stimulated by an action potential the sacs merge with the cell membrane releasing the neurotransmitter into the synapse where it drifts across. If the neurotransmitter docks with a receptor it then stimulates an action potential in the receptor cell. Having sufficient vesicle activity is essential for healthy brain function. Animal studies show us that omega-3 deficiency lowers vesicle density in the hippocampus, the area of the brain central to learning and memory, by 30 per cent, significantly reducing the ability of these brain cells to function optimally.

Synaptic pruning

The end of a nerve cell looks a bit like the branches of a tree: there is the main stem (axon) and then the branches (axon terminal). In general, more connections (or branches) mean more reliable communication in a neural network. However, sometimes there can be too many branches. Excess connections can make communication in the brain less efficient or disordered. So, at various stages during development the brain undertakes a process called synaptic pruning, clearing away any unnecessary branches. Sometimes this pruning process goes awry. Like an overzealous gardener who cuts too many branches off a young sapling. Excessive pruning is a problem and has been associated with increased risk of schizophrenia, for example.

Omega-3-deficient diets cause excessive pruning, change the shape of the hippocampus and impair spatial working memory in animal models.

Brain cell survival

Brain cells incur damage with use and aging. Compounds called growth factors help protect brain cells, stimulate neurogenesis and repair damage. DHA increases the expression of key growth factors.

Gene expression

DHA increases the activity of genes involved in neuroplasticity, learning and the maturation of brain cells. Conversely, DHA deficiency during pregnancy and in the perinatal period is associated with genetic changes linked to increased brain cell death and neurodegeneration. A study in which 174 Alzheimer's disease (AD) patients were randomly assigned to receive either 1.7g DHA and 0.6g EPA or a placebo daily, six months of omega-3 supplementation led to differential gene expression, including the upregulation of genes that code for proteins linked to cell signalling, protection against AD and neurodegeneration, and several that play a role in regulating inflammation.

Inflammation

Inflammation refers to the activity of the immune system in response to infection, illness or injury. Immune cells that travel in the bloodstream have receptors on their surfaces that recognise pathogens. If the cells come into contact with a harmful microorganism they release chemical messengers in the form of proteins called cytokines. These molecules alert nearby immune cells of the threat and augment local tissues. For example by making their membranes more permeable to allow more microbe-fighting immune cells in. Cytokines are an essential part of a healthy and effective immune response. However, in excess or over prolonged periods their actions can have negative downstream consequences with deleterious effects on mood and mental health.

It had been thought that once the microbe had been thwarted and the threat eliminated, the inflammatory response would simply 'ease off', like the way a fire burns itself out when it runs out of fuel. However, it is now known that the resolution of inflammation is an active process, like the active step you have to take to turn off a light after you have turned it on. Switching off inflammation requires a special group of molecules that are collectively called specialised pro-resolving mediators:

- **Resolvins** – Derived from EPA and DHA, resolvins reduce inflammation, lower inflammatory pain, repair damaged tissues and remove neutrophils (white blood cells, the main constituents of pus).
- **Protectins** – Derived from DHA, protectins protect retinal and neuronal cells from a type of cell death that is triggered by oxidative stress.
- **Maresins** – Produced by white blood cells and derived from DHA, maresins reduce inflammation, promote wound healing and help to resolve allergic reactions.

Oxidative stress

Have you ever walked around a gallery and seen a group of children on a school trip? Draped in hi-vis vests the accompanying adults often have the children hold hands and walk in pairs, the added layer of oversight (each child's buddy) helping to keep the group organised. Without this system each child is liable to run off, attach itself to another group, or get up to mischief in some other way. Free radicals – aka reactive oxygen species (ROS) – are molecules that contain an atom of oxygen and an uneven number of electrons. To a degree they are not a problem; ROS are signalling molecules in their own right and play a role in wound healing. However, in excess and unchecked, these unpartnered electrons can 'run off', attach themselves to other molecules and get up to biological mischief. This process is called oxidation and, at the harmful end, it creates 'oxidative stress', which is linked to inflammation, accelerated aging and illness.

Its high level of unsaturation makes DHA prone to oxidation. That is, the free radicals take up the spare seats at DHA's table and interfere with its activity. And, unfortunately, the high metabolic activity of the brain makes it a very pro-oxidation environment. This, obviously, sounds like a recipe for disaster. But here's the cool part: DHA dials up the production of antioxidants, especially in the hippocampus, one of the brain areas most damaged in Alzheimer's disease.

So DHA is the cornerstone of brain development and the availability of preformed DHA may well have been the driving force behind the development not just of our well-connected brains but of the complex thought and culture that emerges from them. Indeed, brain DHA concentration is highest in the PFC, the region of the brain that coordinates our higher functions. With such a high concentration of DHA in the brain you would expect either that we would be able to synthesise it, or for this fat to be abundant in the environment. If we need so much of it, it would make sense that there was enough of it to go around. But that's not quite the case.

The omega-3 fats are essential, meaning we must attain them from dietary sources to build, sustain and protect our large brains. However, most of the omega-3 present in plant foods is ALA and our conversion of ALA to DHA is limited; it is highly unlikely that our consumption of plants was able to supply enough. Some theorists have tried to plug this biochemical gap by suggesting that humans attained our DHA from eating the meat and brains of other animals. This degree of brain consumption also seems unlikely because this level of hunting would require huge amounts of energy. It would be unsustainable. The incompatibility of this theory with the biological reality of our brains indicates that, for a significant period of our evolutionary development, we had ready access to abundant preformed DHA. So where on earth did it come from?

Off the Savannah and into the Sea

If we take a look at brain size through human evolution you can see (below) the steady increase in cranial volume.

Mean Brain Volumes and Encephalisation Quotients (EQ) for Selected Hominoid Species

Species	Brain volume (cm³)	EQ
Australopithecus afarensis	384	1.45
A. africanus	420	1.62
A. boisei	488	1.72
A. robustus	502	1.92
Homo habilis	579–597	2.10–2.29
H. rudolfensis	709	2.11
H. erectus	820–844	2.38–2.44
H. sapiens	1,250	4.26

Australopithecus, a genus of hominin and an ancestor to the *Homo* human species, lived in eastern and southern Africa around 4.2 million years ago. The brain volume of land-dwelling *Australopithecus* remained at a comparatively modest 400–500cm³ through its roughly 3-million-year existence. *Homo habilis*, who emerged from *Australopithecus* 2.3–2.8 million years ago, had a brain volume of around 600cm³. *Homo sapiens* (us) have a brain volume of about 1,300cm³. In contrast to the *Australopithecus* years, brain size between *Homo habilis* and *Homo sapiens* doubled in just 1 million years. The question is: what accounts for the speed of this growth, particularly in light of the high energy demands of brain tissue?

In the movie *Cast Away*, Chuck Noland, played by Tom Hanks, is marooned on an uninhabited island in the Pacific Ocean following a plane crash. Stranded with only items salvaged from the wreckage of the plane, he has to learn how to fend for himself for what is eventually four years. He is shown surviving mainly on coconuts, fish, crab and rainwater.

The familiar image of our early ancestors is of small nomadic tribes living on largely arid plains, subsisting on wild game, insects and a variety of plants. Some propose that increased consumption of energy-rich meat or starchy tubers contributed to human brain expansion.

However, contemporary evidence suggests that, like Chuck, access to water and, in particular, seafood was key to our survival and perhaps even the defining feature of our modern *Homo sapiens* brain because it gave us abundant access to preformed DHA. EPA and DHA are synthesised in aquatic environments by microalgae. When fish and other sea animals consume this algae, they accumulate EPA and DHA in their tissues. When we eat fish and seafood we absorb these preformed EPA and DHA fats.

It seems likely that the image of early modern humans as mainly land-dwelling creatures is incorrect and that for many generations our ancestors were lakeshore- or coastal-dwelling. For example, bone fossil analysis shows that, compared to the Neanderthals, seafood was a staple food for early modern humans, making up between 10–50 per cent of the diet depending on location.

This shift to the inclusion and reliance on freshwater and marine seafoods in the diet correlates with the development of more complex human culture. Strikingly, it also corresponds with an increased volume of grey matter in the brain. Grey matter refers to the cell bodies of neurones and glial cells, as well as synapses, the points of communication between brain cells. The more points of connection and communication in a system, the greater the level of computation and the more complex that system becomes. You will see in the next chapter how this effect plays out on the individual level too – how DHA availability affects foetal brain development.

With an expensive brain to fuel, a diet rich in seafood had two key advantages for our ancestors:

First is the lower effort-to-reward ratio. Persistence in the hunting of larger animals requires many individuals tracking an animal for a long period of time, using a significant amount of energy. In contrast, fish, which are a rich source of nutrients, vitamins and minerals, can be speared, netted or caught by hand with much less effort and energy expenditure. Other important marine foods include mussels, clams, oysters and scallops. Mussels grow attached to rocks, making them particularly easy to collect. Others like scallops can propel themselves through the water but move slowly and can easily be collected by hand from the shallows. These foods, which are also a source of easily digestible protein, could safely be eaten raw but also cook very quickly, requiring less fuel for cooking.

Secondly, and crucially, these foods are incredibly rich in pre-formed long-chain omega-3 fats. One 140g serving of mackerel provides sufficient omega-3 for an adult for a week (this figure is based on the amount required to reduce the risk of heart disease – 500mg per day of EPA and DHA); 100g of crab supplies nearly half of an adult's weekly omega-3 requirement. At least Chuck's brain was well nourished.

In addition, the omega-3 in seafood comes packaged with other brain-healthy essential nutrients, vitamins and minerals, many of which work in synergy with EPA and DHA to build and protect the brain. A 100g serving of oysters provides nearly all of an adult's daily requirement of vitamin D, and more than 100 per cent of zinc, selenium and vitamin B12. Mussels are also rich in brain-healthy vitamin B12, iron, zinc, selenium and iodine. Coincidentally, these nutrients are essential for your body to produce the enzyme that protects fatty acids from oxidative damage. You'll hear how these nutrients work together to protect the brain in later chapters.

Conclusion

The evolution of body size is a feature of protein availability. But brain size and connectivity depend on the availability of a few very special fats. That is, the limiting factor for the growth of the human brain is the availability of preformed omega-3 fat. The large brains of modern humans were fed with irreplaceable preformed omega-3 from marine and aquatic sources. These fats are absolutely essential to the structural integrity and proper functioning of our brains. In a sense they made us who we are. Consequently, we continue, in our modern food environments, to require a regular intake of these preformed long-chain fatty acids. This is where the evidence becomes very troubling. In the UK, instead of the recommended 1–2 portions of oily fish per week, most adults are consuming around a portion per month. Even more worrying are the very low rates of fatty fish consumption in children. According to a survey published in 2017 only 4.5 per cent of children in the UK were meeting the oily fish consumption recommendation. Available evidence suggests this shortfall is not being rectified through supplementation; it is much more likely that we are facing a situation in which almost no UK children are getting adequate amounts of these essential fats. On top of that, other components of our diets directly compete with the conversion of omega-3s and limit their uptake. The question is: what impact might this be having on brain development, cognition and mental health?

The decline in essential fatty acid consumption is, I think, a significant contributing factor to the increased vulnerability of our brains to the stresses of life, but as I noted earlier, the brain needs a range of different materials for healthy growth and maintenance. Vitamins, minerals, phytochemicals (from plants), the by-products of bacterial fermentation of polyphenols (plant compounds beneficial to human health) and fibre (also from plants) all play crucial roles in brain and mental health. A minimally processed diet, rich in leafy green veg, wholegrains, nuts, seafood and so on used to provide these nutrients in abundance. Almost anywhere humans migrated in the world these foods nourished our remarkable brains. However, like invasive plants that once introduced crowd out and kill off native species, the modern ultra-processed, industrialised, Western-style diet is killing traditional dietary patterns and simultaneously depriving our brains of their essential building blocks. The consequence is increased prevalence of neurodevelopmental and neurodegenerative illness, as we shall see.

For some other essential nutrients like vitamin C the signs of deficiency show up very quickly, and, when they do, those signs are dramatic – swollen, bleeding gums and bruised skin are hard to ignore. And the rapidity of recovery following treatment ensures that, for any observer, the importance of vitamin C for physical health is obvious. However, unlike bruises and loose teeth, the signs of brain nutrient insufficiency are much more subtle and take much longer to emerge; there is no dramatic before-and-after that would make the effects of low intake apparent. In addition, the inaccessibility of the brain makes experiments incredibly difficult to conduct. Nonetheless, the totality of evidence from population observation, cell experiments, animal trials and clinical studies paints a disturbing picture. Our worsening diets and high population levels of nutritional deficiency are contributing to lower IQs, increasing rates of developmental disorders, impaired emotional regulation, poorer stress resilience, neurodegeneration and worse mental health.

Our diet gave us our beautiful brains and now it is destroying them. And the risk starts, as we'll see in the next chapter, before we're even conceived.

PART II

BUILDING BABY'S BRAIN – THE NUTRIENTS REQUIRED FOR BRAIN DEVELOPMENT . . . THAT WE'RE NOT GETTING

CHAPTER 3

THE MATERNAL UNIVERSE

AS A CHILD I had something of an obsession with the periodic table. What captivated me most was that I was *made of these elements*. These tiny, invisible particles that could be neatly arranged in a table were the very stuff of life. Not only that, but those elements were forged in stars. For a child who was prone to spending a lot of time staring at the sky it was thrilling to learn that I was made of such distant material. To think that parts of me (or what was to become me) travelled hundreds of millions of miles through space to coalesce, come to life, develop consciousness and be able to reflect on its own existence is a feature of the human brain that is still capable of making me feel woozy with awe.

A microcosm of this astonishing process occurs with every pregnancy. This time, though, instead of being composed of the debris of exploding stars, the elements that make up the developing foetus are microscopic fragments of the mother's diet. Amino acids – the building blocks of proteins – broken down from baked beans or a piece of cheese, might become part of a muscle or skin cell. Fats from a fried egg will find their way into the foetal brain and retina. In this way we can take the familiar 'you are what you eat' back a step: you are what your mother ate (and in some cases what your grandmother ate; more on that later).

This, of course, means that what the mother eats in preparation for and during her pregnancy is of great importance to the development of the foetus both in relation to growth and later health risks. Pregnant women are cautioned against drinking alcohol because, depending on the amount and frequency, its consumption can lead to low birth weight, learning difficulties, memory problems, and attention- and hyperactivity-related conditions. It is also common knowledge that an excess of vitamin A can cause malformation of the foetal head, brain, spinal cord and heart, which is why pregnant women are advised to avoid eating liver, a very rich source of retinol vitamin A. However, most people do not know about how the availability of other nutrients contributes to the brain development and future mental health of children, beginning at preconception. Maternal and paternal nutrition quality *before* conception has lifelong effects on the health of the child. And the state of a woman's health at the point of conception has an important impact on the health of her child and subsequent generations.

According to a review on the links between maternal diet and child health published in the *Lancet* in 2018, the Western diet is typically deficient in key nutrients for brain development like magnesium (see page 209), iodine and folate. In the UK, 77 per cent of young women (aged 18–25) have lower than recommended intakes of iodine, and 96 per cent had iron and folate intakes lower than those recommended for healthy pregnancy. Let's look at each of these in turn.

Folate

Of all the nutrients known to be important for a healthy pregnancy and the development of a healthy nervous system, folate tends to be the one that most people have heard of. Folate is a B vitamin found in leafy green vegetables like spinach, veg from the brassica family like cabbage, broccoli and Brussels sprouts, beans and legumes, wholegrains and fortified foods. It can be difficult to attain the recommended amounts of folate from the diet so supplementation with its synthetic form – folic acid – is advised. Adequate folate intake prevents neural tube defects such as spina bifida, where an opening in the spine from early foetal development does not close properly. Folate also helps to protect the health of the mother, reducing the risk of pre-eclampsia, a potentially fatal pregnancy condition that can cause organ damage, for which the only cure is to deliver the baby.

Folic acid/folate is required in such high concentrations during pregnancy that over 80 countries around the world mandate that common foods should be fortified with it to reduce the risk of neural tube defects. Cases of and deaths from spina bifida have reduced in the US since grain fortification was introduced. This is an important example of the impact of industrialised foods on child development (folate is stripped from the grain during refining) and the appropriate introduction of food policy to address the identified risks. A recent UK review has concluded that white (but not wholemeal) flour in the UK should be fortified with folic acid.

However, most people are not made aware that the neural tube (which becomes the brain and spinal cord) begins to develop early in pregnancy and therefore folate should be taken *before* conception to ensure that levels are adequate from the moment of conception. In a study of 1.5 million women in China, those who took folate supplements for three months before they became pregnant had lower rates of miscarriage, preterm birth, low birth weight, stillbirth, birth defects, face malformations and neonatal death compared to those who did not supplement early. Folic acid supplementation throughout pregnancy also seems to improve child cognition at age seven compared to women who only took the nutrient during the first trimester (as is generally recommended in the UK).

The thing about folate (like vitamin C) is that the consequences of deficiency are overt. What about all of the nutrients that are persistently deficient in the general population where the negative outcomes are less obvious, or take longer to develop, but are no less severe in terms of their impact on brain and mental health across the lifespan?

Iodine

Iodine is one of the most important nutrients for brain development that we never talk about. Rich sources of iodine are seaweed, fish and seafood. It is also added to animal feed, so our other main dietary sources are dairy, eggs and (outside the UK) iodised salt. For this reason, a range of studies report that omnivores typically meet or exceed the adequate intake for iodine. Vegetarians have moderate to low amounts but vegans hover around 20–30 per cent of the adequate intake.

It's also required for the production of thyroid hormone, low levels of which (hypothyroidism) can slow the metabolism, leading to tiredness, fatigue and weight gain in adults. But normal levels of thyroid hormone are also essential for brain development, where it determines neural network density. So much so that the World Health Organization (WHO) describes iodine deficiency as 'the single most important preventable cause of brain damage' worldwide. At the extreme, iodine deficiency during pregnancy leads to a condition in children called cretinism, in which physical and mental development are severely impaired. However, less severe iodine deficiency is linked to intellectual and cognitive deficits across populations. 'In an iodine-deficient population, everybody may seem to be slow and rather sleepy. The quality of life is poor, ambition is blunted, and the community becomes trapped in a self-perpetuating cycle,' the WHO explains. They note that people who live in areas of iodine deficiency have IQs up to 13.5 points lower than peers in non-deficient areas. But we're not talking about obscure isolated communities. Iodine deficiency was relatively common and widespread in America until the 1920s when iodised salt was introduced. Researchers have used this as an opportunity to analyse the impact of iodine availability during pregnancy on child outcomes. They compared children born before (1920–23), during (1924–27) and after (1928–31) iodisation, following them across their working lives. Those born after iodisation had better educational attainment, were significantly more likely to be employed and earned 11 per cent more than those born before iodine was introduced. This is why the widespread iodine deficiency in the UK in women of childbearing age is such a concern when thinking about the brain health of the next generation. Low population intake means that whole groups of children will not be reaching their full cognitive potential.

The Avon Longitudinal Study of Parents and Children (ALSPAC) is a cohort study following the health of thousands of children born in

1991 and 1992 in the former county of Avon in England. The study provides a rich database of information on a range of health and life outcomes. One research team analysed the cognitive outcomes of the children of 958 women as a function of the mother's iodine status during the first trimester of pregnancy. The cut-off value for sufficient urinary iodine is 150µg per gram. So, the first thing to note is the high level of insufficiency – 67 per cent of the women in this group had a urinary iodine concentration lower than this, indicating mild to moderate deficiency. *Deficiency was the norm* and none of the women reported supplementing with iodine or consuming iodine during pregnancy.

Impact of Maternal Iodine Deficiency on the Iodine Status of Avon-based Children Born between 1991 and 1992

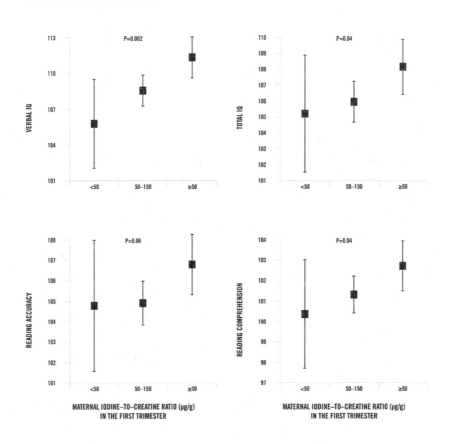

The researchers conclude: 'Low maternal iodine status was associated with an increased risk of suboptimum scores for verbal IQ at age 8 years, and reading accuracy, comprehension, and reading score at age 9 years, even after adjustment for many potential confounders. Furthermore, our results suggest a worsening trend in cognitive outcome with decreasing maternal iodine status.' In the previous graph you can see a linear relationship between maternal iodine and several cognitive outcomes in the children.

I find this really worrying because the negative effects of iodine insufficiency during gestation, when the brain is being built, are irreversible. Insufficient iodine in the first 14 weeks of pregnancy permanently suppresses child IQ.

In their iodine factsheet the British Dietetic Association states that, like folic acid, 'you should make sure you have been having enough [iodine] in your diet for several months before getting pregnant'. However, it is not clear that this message is getting across. In an opportunity sample of my social media audience (93 per cent female, largest age group 25–34), while many were told to supplement with folic acid in the first trimester, none mentioned iodine.

However, it is not just for children's sake that we should be concerned about iodine insufficiency in the general population. In a recent analysis of over 7,000 Taiwanese elders (average age 75), those with dementia were significantly more likely to have had hypothyroidism. Specifically, 0.9 per cent of those with dementia had hypothyroidism. In people without dementia it was 0.4 per cent.

I know that this figure seems tiny, and no, by itself, hypothyroidism isn't driving dementia. However, we understand that dementia is a multifactorial condition, with risk factors that accumulate and compound over time, until they reach a tipping point. For some people, the development of hypothyroidism will be the factor that tips them over that point.

Conception

And finally, a special mention for both brain cells and the development of blood vessels. Healthy, well-distributed and properly functioning blood vessels are the framework of a well-organised, properly supplied brain. And these foundations are laid in the first moments of conception. The very first cells to differentiate are those of the endothelium, the cells that line the blood vessels (capillaries, veins and arteries). The vascular system forms the scaffolding for the brain (with many miles of blood vessels) and the cardiovascular system. Additionally, the placenta is a highly vascular structure, specialised in filtering the maternal blood to supply nutrients and limiting its exposure to toxins. An important nutrient required at this stage is a fatty acid called arachidonic acid (ARA).

Arachidonic acid can be converted from linolenic acid; however, during foetal development it seems to be important to have access to preformed ARA. Food sources of ARA include sardines, salmon, eggs, chicken, pork, beef and dairy. The only significant plant source of ARA is seaweed.

Alongside DHA, arachidonic acid helps to maintain the fluidity of cell membranes, with additional roles in cell signalling and receptor function. ARA is a precursor to a class of compounds with roles in the regulation of inflammation, immunity and proper functioning of the brain's reward system. Arachidonic acid remains important during adulthood, comprising approximately 10 per cent of the total fatty acids in the adult brain. The distribution of the important fat and its essential role in vascular differentiation and development give further support to the central role of seafood in our evolutionary progress.

For optimal brain development certain nutrients need to be available from the moment of conception. Of course, not all conceptions are planned. Some of us have the dubious honour of being a 'happy accident'. However, many conceptions are planned. For example, when a woman comes off her hormonal contraception in advance of trying to conceive. And with more women and couples delaying starting a family due to social factors (such as housing and childcare costs) it is likely to increasingly be the case. Therefore, it is important that prospective parents understand the importance of preconception nutrition for a healthy pregnancy, optimal infant brain development and future health.

A TALE OF TWO BRAINS

Yasmin is a 31-year-old British woman. Her mother, Eleni, was Greek and had grown up eating home-cooked food and this is what she prepared for Yasmin. Hortopita – a pie made with greens and feta – vine leaves stuffed with rice and vegetables, courgette fritters, taramasalata, hummus. Raised Catholic, Eleni also maintained the tradition of eating fish every Friday. Each meal came with a simple green salad dressed with vinegar and olive oil, and usually some bread from the bakery too. The family could not afford to eat out so they rarely had takeaways; besides, Eleni didn't trust the food from most fast-food vendors. '*Myrízei períerga*,' she would say – 'it smells strange'. Though she sometimes felt different not eating the same foods as her school friends, the result was that Yasmin grew up with a taste for fresh, simply cooked foods. And this is the food she would make for herself. On nights where she really did not have the energy to cook, she would buy some bread rolls, hummus, olives and marinated anchovies from the supermarket on the way home and promise herself she would try to cook something at the weekend.

Zoe, also 31, grew up on the border of Essex and east London. Her mother, Pat, was a warm woman who doted on her daughter. Her favourite part of the day was when they would sit around their tiny kitchen table and have dinner while Zoe talked about school. She made Zoe's favourite, oven chips, chicken nuggets and baked beans, at least once a week. On other days she would have mini pizzas, jacket potatoes with cheese, or tuna pasta bake. Zoe liked sweetcorn and peas (with ketchup) but could not be persuaded to eat much other veg. They drank orange or blackcurrant squash. On a Friday Pat would treat them both to an iced finger.

When Zoe started working and cooking for herself, time was the main priority. Pasta and a jar of sauce was a regular fallback, along with beans on toast. She still enjoyed the flavours she grew up with, like pasta salad, and was partial to the occasional sausage sandwich. On days when she felt guilty for not eating much veg, she would make a chicken stir-fry with black bean or sweet and sour sauce. And an iced finger (or a chocolate éclair, if she was feeling fancy) on Friday nights.

When they became pregnant, her habitual diet meant that Yasmin had higher blood levels of most B vitamins, magnesium and ARA, EPA and DHA than Zoe. Because a woman's nutritional status in the weeks before and around conception lay the foundation for the early development of the blood vessels that will form the foetus and the placenta, this meant that Yasmin's baby had stronger nutritional foundations for brain development. Additionally, women who eat a Mediterranean-style (minimally processed) diet are less likely to develop gestational diabetes (see page 94), which is a risk factor for preterm birth. Her higher intake of refined, low-fibre foods with added sugars meant that Zoe's blood sugar was elevated towards the end of her pregnancy, though happily this did not tip over into gestational diabetes. The mothers' diets during pregnancy also began to shape their children's taste preferences, as you will read in chapter 15.

Chapter 4

THE IMPORTANCE OF DHA

GHERKINS. ICE CREAM. Pizza. These are some of the most commonly reported foods craved during pregnancy. Many theories have been proposed as to why so many pregnant women (50–90 per cent) report craving specific foods. A popular hypothesis is that the woman craves foods containing the nutrients needed in greater quantities during pregnancy; that the craving is the way the body asks for what it needs. However, this idea comes unstuck when you consider that most of the nutrients beneficial for the developing foetus and pregnant woman can be found more abundantly in beans and leafy greens than fast food and cake. It looks more likely that these 'cravings' are driven by social expectations and cultural norms. Women grow up being told to expect pregnancy cravings, it becomes part of the shared experience of pregnancy, and they are therefore more likely to attribute subsequent food desire to the pregnancy.

My mother said that she craved sardines when she was pregnant with me, and I certainly recall that sardine sandwiches (tinned sardines, mashed, and mixed with chopped onion) were a regular snack when I was growing up. If pregnancy cravings really were about responding to increased nutrient demand, then her sardine cravings would make a lot of sense because a woman's DHA requirement increases during pregnancy, especially during the third trimester, and cold-water oily fish such as sardines are a great source. My mother, by the way, had no idea about this. It was just cheap and tasty. Little did she know that this rather humble snack was contributing to my brain development.

In fact, the mother's body preferentially pulls these fats out of her diet and stores and delivers them to the developing foetus. One of the world's leading researchers on the importance of essential fats for brain development, Professor Michael Crawford, describes this process as the 'biomagnification' of DHA. Imagine I give you a handful of marbles. Most of them are clear, just plain glass. But one in every ten of them is red because at the centre is a ruby. You would be inclined to pick out and keep the valuable red marbles and discard the rest. Then I give you another handful of marbles. After a while you would have a good collection of precious red marbles – you will have preferentially kept hold of them because you know they are valuable. This 'preferential transport' is what the body and in particular the foetal brain does with preformed DHA from the mother's blood. Precious DHA is selectively incorporated into these vital tissues. Interestingly, the reverse is also true: the foetal compartment *rejects the ARA and DHA precursor fats (linolenic acid and alpha-linolenic acid)*. It doesn't want to make them itself, there is no time for that. So the precursors are returned to the mother's bloodstream. Like the plain marbles, they are discarded.

It's hard to overstate the evolutionary implications of this process. These fats are so absolutely fundamental and irreplaceable that the maternal body evolved mechanisms to make, extract and then deliver and concentrate them in the foetal brain. Our bodies are telling us how important these nutrients are, yet, with some studies showing that 92 per cent of pregnant women are deficient, expectant mothers are not routinely advised to consume enough oily fish or to supplement with omega-3 during pregnancy. I honestly don't understand why. Perhaps it's because, unlike folate deficiency, DHA deficiency doesn't result in an open wound. But surely we don't need children to endure that level of physical insult for the government to act on established science?

So, for the avoidance of doubt, let's look at just some of the essential functions of DHA, from premature birth to child IQ. By the end of this chapter you'll understand why I find it so worrying that less than 5 per cent of UK children are getting enough.

Prematurity

In the last 12 weeks of pregnancy the brain more than doubles in size and accelerates its accumulation of DHA, particularly in the prefrontal cortex, the area of the brain that manages and coordinates complex behaviour. Accumulation continues up to around the age of two. This means that the mother's diet during pregnancy and breastfeeding is crucial to the availability of preformed DHA (and DPA, an intermediary fatty acid that can be converted into DHA) for the developing infant.

This rapid development of the brain during the last 2–3 months of pregnancy underlies some of the risk associated with being born prematurely. A preterm or premature birth is one that occurs before 37 weeks. The World Health Organization defines the subcategories of preterm birth as:

- Extremely preterm (less than 28 weeks)
- Very preterm (28–32 weeks)
- Moderate to late preterm (32–37 weeks)

Others define an 'early birth' as one that occurs before 37 weeks and a 'very early birth' means a baby that is born before 34 weeks' gestation.

Being born early presents a range of risks and complications for the baby. Common physical risks include heart and breathing problems, poor kidney function and increased risk of infection. But there is compelling evidence of long-term psychological risks for babies who are born before 37 weeks. A joint study conducted by two prestigious research facilities, King's College London and Sweden's Karolinska Institute, uncovered an association between being born early and psychiatric illness in adulthood. To do this they looked at the health data of over 1 million Swedes born between 1973 and 1985, who were still living in

Sweden at age 16. They found that, compared to people born 'to term' – between 37 and 41 weeks – those born between 32 and 36 weeks were:

- 1.6 times more likely to have psychosis.
- 1.3 times more likely to have major depression.
- 2.7 times more likely to have bipolar disorder.

And those born before 32 weeks were:

- 2.5 times more likely to have psychosis.
- 2.9 times more likely to have major depression.
- 7.4 times more likely to have bipolar disorder.

This increased risk was independent of known risk factors for these outcomes, such as socioeconomic status and the mother's mental health. Low birth weight is an associated feature of preterm birth that comes with its own risks, including a higher incidence of autism.

There are a number of reasons for these outcomes. First is simply that the baby's nervous system has not had enough time to mature and is exposed to the outside world far too soon. Another important factor is the way that premature birth restricts the access and opportunity for parental care.

The foetus starts to develop body fat in the third trimester, from around week 29 of pregnancy. This fat is essential for keeping the baby warm. When adults become cold their bodies automatically trigger the shiver reflex. These rapid automatic muscle contractions help to generate heat, protecting the body from hypothermia. However, babies are unable to shiver. Instead, they stay warm by burning fat. Babies that are born early will have limited fat deposits to keep them warm and may need to go into an incubator, a heated, transparent chamber that manages the temperature for premature babies. Incubators no doubt have saved millions of lives but the cost incurred is that parents are less able to hold their babies. These early moments of physical contact and emotional connection help to regulate the baby's stress system and initiate some features of neural development.

Preterm birth may also mean that the mother is unwell and in need of urgent or prolonged care, which may keep her separated from her new baby. Skin-to-skin contact between mother and baby has been shown to reduce the baby's cortisol; separation increases the baby's experience of stress.

The parents of babies born prematurely are also likely to be very worried and distressed, concerned about the health of the baby and perhaps also the mother, and mourning the temporary loss of the parenting role as the care of the baby is necessarily assumed by hospital staff. Stressed parents may subsequently find it more difficult to regulate or soothe their babies. For example, they may be hypervigilant for signs of illness and find it hard to relax. Some preterm babies will also have additional needs, especially around feeding, which can make it difficult to settle into a routine when the family goes home.

These neuropsychological risks reduce with increased birth weight and gestational age. That is to say that the closer to term a baby can be born, the better for its long-term physical and mental health. While the risk factors for premature delivery are diverse and not entirely controllable (see box on page 54) there is one surprisingly simple way to reduce the risk of a baby being born before 37 weeks. Pregnant women who have a higher intake of omega-3 fats during pregnancy have a longer gestation. This means that babies are more likely to be born to term, rather than prematurely.

A recent Cochrane Review showed that increased intake of omega-3 fatty acids during pregnancy reduced the risk of a baby being born before 37 weeks by 11 per cent and before 34 weeks by 42 per cent.

I want to be very careful here. I am, of course, not suggesting that all premature births are preventable, nor that a premature delivery should be attributed to the dietary choices of individual women. There are many complex causes of preterm birth and in many cases it is simply not possible to identify a cause. However, the Cochrane Review concludes that there is 'high-quality evidence' for a simple nutritional intervention, 'omega-3 supplementation' being an effective strategy for reducing the incidence of preterm birth.

Risk Factors for Premature Delivery

The list of risk factors of preterm birth include:

- Health of mother – the presence of diabetes or hypertension
- Pregnancy resulting from IVF treatment
- Age of mother
  - Women younger than 18 are at higher risk
  - Women over the age of 35 either because they are more likely to have the health risk factors mentioned above or to have used IVF treatment
- Smoking
- Alcohol intake
- Stress
- Lack of social support
- Working a job that requires many hours of standing
- Being from an ethnic minority background

Many of these features overlap with poverty. We will come back to this in the chapter on the role of nutrition in the cycle of poverty.

The review found that the optimum dose was between 500mg and 1,000mg of omega-3 per day (of which at least 500mg should be DHA) from the end of the first trimester (12 weeks). Given this recommendation and the established low consumption of omega-3 fats in the UK population, it is surprising and disappointing that most commercially available supplements in the UK that are designed for use during pregnancy (rather than preconception or during breastfeeding) do not contain sufficient omega-3 fats. Of those that do the levels are lower than recommended by the Cochrane group as of October 2022.

A Breakdown of the Recommended Intake of Omega-3 in Commercially Available Supplements

Product	DHA (mg per recommended serving)
Active Iron Pregnancy Plus	250
Bassetts Vitamins During Pregnancy Strawberry & Orange Flavour Pastilles	40
Boots Pregnancy Essential Vitamins	0
Proceive Pregnancy Supplement Trimester 1	0
Proceive Pregnancy Supplement Trimester 2	0
Proceive Pregnancy Supplement Trimester 3	0
Seven Seas Pregnancy Vitamins with Folic Acid	0
Viridian Pregnancy Complex	0
Vitabiotics Pregnacare Original	0
Vitabiotics Pregnacare Max	300
Vitabiotics Pregnacare Plus Omega-3	300

In addition, the review found there was moderate-quality evidence for the protective role of omega-3s on reduced perinatal death, fewer neonatal care admissions and low birth weight. This should make us think seriously about population dietary habits and the nutritional advice given to women during conception and pregnancy.

On that note, in August 2022, I emailed two UK organisations well placed to advise women on the importance of omega-3 in pregnancy, the Royal College of Obstetricians and Gynaecologists (RCOG), and the pregnancy charity, Tommy's. I asked whether they had any plans to make a statement regarding the Cochrane recommendations.

Tommy's told me that my email had been forwarded to the 'Pregnancy Information team to find out whether they're currently developing any additional guidance on nutrition covering these areas'. As of November 2022, I have not heard from the Pregnancy Information team.

The RCOG said: 'The RCOG does not currently have a guideline specific to this topic; however, our update to Green-top Guideline no.

31 *Investigation and Care of a Small-for-Gestational-Age Fetus and a Growth Restricted Fetus* does mention omega-3. I anticipate the guideline will be published in the first half of next year.

'NICE [National Institute for Health and Care Excellence] are currently doing an update of Public Health guideline [PH11] Maternal and child nutrition, which may cover this.' I read the final scope document of the PH11 guideline, which is due for publication in November 2023. It makes no mention of omega-3s.

In addition, the NHS advice pages 'Vitamins, supplements and nutrition in pregnancy', 'Have a heathy diet in pregnancy' and 'Vegetarian or vegan and pregnant' do not reference omega-3 fats. So, despite research evidence being clear on the essential need for adequate omega-3 intake during pregnancy, this information is absent from official government pregnancy health recommendations.

PRETERM BIRTH AND DONOR BREAST MILK

Mothers of babies who are born very preterm may not yet be lactating, so their babies, before 32 weeks, are fed with donor breast milk. Compared to formula at this age, breast milk reduces the risk of the baby developing necrotising enterocolitis (NEC), a very serious illness in which inflammation can kill tissue in the baby's colon. Very sick, very small and usually premature babies are at greatest risk of NEC. Doctors are not sure exactly what causes NEC; however, there is thought to be a relationship with oxidative stress. Unfortunately, many of the interventions required to save the lives of very preterm babies, such as blood transfusions, oxygen therapy and total parenteral nutrition, increase oxidative stress.

Research by Dr Simon Dyall has shown that very preterm babies are not receiving the right type and amounts of fatty acids on neonatal units. Preterm babies are receiving too much linolenic acid and insufficient ARA and DHA. Donor milk was found to have low levels of ARA and almost no DHA. Donor milk was also found to have higher markers of oxidative damage

---

to the fatty acids. The research group have made recommendations to milk banks regarding the treatment and storage of donated breast milk (such as storing it in dark-coloured bottles and limiting its exposure to light) to help protect the fatty acid profile. But what about the donors themselves?

Women who donate breast milk to support at-risk babies are doing a wonderful thing. However, in the UK there are currently no recommendations for what women who donate their breast milk should eat, which feels like a huge oversight when we are talking about the nutrition of the most vulnerable babies. They should be supported in engaging in behaviours that can help to improve the health and outcomes not only of the recipients but also their own babies and even themselves. For example, evidence shows that short-term changes in dietary DHA and EPA increase their levels in breast milk. A Brazilian study found that supplying nursing mothers with around 100g of sardines 2–3 times per week increased the levels of DPA and DHA in her milk.

After 32 weeks preterm babies are fed using formula. This may be in the form of a powder that is mixed with water or a pre-mixed liquid. Again, Simon Dyall's group wanted to assess the fatty acid composition and stability of the formula. They found some variation in actual nutrient content compared to the manufacturers' listed nutritional composition. Most of the nutrients varied within reasonable boundaries; however, they found very low levels of ARA. In addition, once opened and exposed to the air, the fatty acids in the powder formula began to oxidise. Liquid formula was observed to be more stable in this regard.

The WHO reports that global rates of premature birth are rising, meaning that more babies across the world are at risk of these physical and mental complications. In the UK 8 per cent of babies are born preterm. This figure is slightly lower than the global average of 10.6 per cent and roughly in line with the other wealthy European countries. However, within countries, women who live in more socioeconomically deprived areas have a higher risk of preterm birth. And this effect is independent of other risk factors. Indeed, poverty is a leading risk factor for preterm birth both inter- and intranationally; there is a higher risk of preterm birth in poor countries and in poorer households in wealthier ones. Poverty affects levels of familial stress, access to healthcare, the type of work a woman is likely to be doing during her pregnancy, the likelihood of being a smoker (the leading preventable cause of prematurity) and, of course, the quality of her diet. Women educated past the age of 16 are more likely to consume their five-a-day than women only educated to 16. Since length of education tends to correlate with earnings, it may be that more educated women are more able to afford a healthier diet.

On the subject of education, perhaps you are wondering about how these brain changes might influence intelligence. Is IQ just a facet of luck? Is it about having 'good genes'? Is the socioeconomic distribution of IQ simply something we have to suck up and deal with? This is – or at the very least it was – the view of a certain Alexander Johnson, Boris to his friends. In 2013 the then Mayor of London (and later British prime minister) gave the annual Margaret Thatcher Lecture for the conservative think-tank, the Centre for Policy Studies. He said:

> *Whatever you may think of the value of IQ tests, it is surely relevant to a conversation about equality that as many as 16 per cent of our species have an IQ below 85, while about 2 per cent have an IQ above 130. The harder you shake the pack, the easier it will be for some cornflakes to get to the top.*
>
> *And for one reason or another . . . the income gap between the top cornflakes and the bottom cornflakes is getting wider than ever. I stress: I don't believe that economic equality is possible; indeed, some measure of inequality is essential for the spirit of envy and keeping up with the Joneses that is, like greed, a valuable spur to economic activity.*

I think he is saying, and I have sense-checked this with others, that: a very small proportion of the population is smart. That wealth, particularly in a competitive economic environment like the UK, is an outcome of IQ, and, therefore, some people are destined to accumulate more wealth than (most) others. And in fact this is good because the (widening) distance between the poor and the wealthy will spur the poor on to work harder.

Not only is this position oxymoronic (if IQ, which is largely fixed, determines social position then no amount of envy or greed will help the poor to shrink that wealth gap), we know that inequality and the 'spirit of envy' is not good for anyone, and is in fact associated with poorer mental health across the whole of society. Moreover, reducing our steep levels of inequality to be more in line with other wealthy nations would reduce mental illness by 5 per cent. He was right about one thing, though: there is a link between IQ and income. So, is there anything we can do to give our children a leg up in the brain game?

Maternal Diet and Child IQ

A study published in the *New England Journal of Medicine* in 2022 looked at the effect of DHA supplementation on the cognitive outcomes of very preterm babies (those born before 29 weeks). Of the study group, 333 babies received the standard nutrition emulsion and 323 had theirs supplemented with 60mg of DHA per kilogram of body weight per day from the first three days of tube feeding until 36 weeks postmenstrual age or home discharge (whichever came first). At five years old the supplemented children had IQs that were on average 3.5 points higher than the unsupplemented group. So, the babies who received DHA in what would have been the last trimester of pregnancy did better cognitively.

We know that DHA accumulation in the brain speeds up in the last trimester, but how might this be linked to IQ? In animal studies, offspring born to mothers that consume diets insufficient in DHA during gestation exhibit reduced neuronal connectivity. One group found a 50 per cent reduction in the connections of mouse hippocampal cells, the area of the brain associated with learning and memory. You can think of connectivity like an exercise in town planning. Imagine that you are designing a new town. There are some key amenities that it is important your residents have access to: a school, a shopping centre, a park, a bank. If you have just one road running between each of these sites, your design is vulnerable. What happens if that road becomes damaged? In that scenario access to that location is greatly diminished if not cut off completely. However, if you design your town to have several routes between each of those destinations then you have some useful back-up options if something goes wrong (see the diagram below).

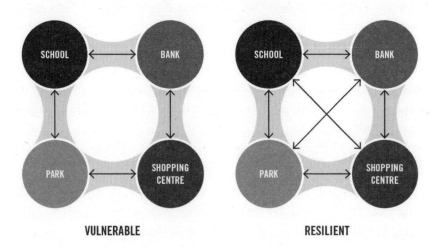

This concept of having additional 'back-up' routes to your destination in case something goes wrong underlies the principle of cognitive reserve that I described in my previous book as the 'pension plan for the brain'. And, like a financial pension plan, the sooner you get started the better. Having 'surplus' neuronal funds provides a cushion against neurodegeneration. However, there is another reason that a high degree of neuronal connectivity might be advantageous: its contribution to IQ.

The measurement of IQ is a contested and controversial discipline in psychology. During my psychology training we learned how culturally irrelevant questions and assessment techniques led to the designation of non-white groups as intellectually inferior, a classification that was used to justify denigration, enslavement and even genocide. Those who endorsed this position reduced IQ to genetic heritability. That is, how much of your intellect has been passed down to you through your genes. Studies of twins and siblings seem to show a high degree of heritability, but the story is complicated. Other than for fixed features like eye colour, genes really tell a story about *potential*. For example, you might have genes that predispose you to being tall, but if you experience malnourishment during childhood your body will not have the substrate, the nutritional building blocks, to grow your body to its full, *genetically determined* potential height. Similarly, a child who inherits the genes that might predispose them to being gifted but whose intellect and curiosity are not recognised or nurtured is unlikely to reach their potential. So genes must interact with the environment to achieve their full potential. Detrimental environmental features will include early life stress, experiences of prejudice, educational and economic exclusion, health inequality and nutrition.

Genes are not the only thing children will *inherit* from their parents: culinary traditions, local food availability and diet quality are also shared features of the child's *in utero* and early life development. A baby may have the genetic potential for a higher IQ, but not receive the adequate nutritional building blocks to fulfil their full promise. This is perhaps evidenced by a disturbing observation in IQ research: global IQ is falling.

The Flynn effect

Named after IQ researcher James Flynn, the Flynn effect is the observation that global IQ consistently increased over the course of the twentieth century. This has been attributed to environmental factors such as better and improved access to education, reduced exposure to toxins such as lead, improved perinatal care and better nutrition. However, since the 1990s Western countries including Norway, Denmark, Australia and Britain have been seeing a decline in IQ. In fact, one report states that high scores in the UK have been 'decimated'. If it were simply that IQ had hit a peak, we would perhaps expect scores to plateau. But decline and 'decimation' indicate that something much more active and worrying has been happening since the 1990s. What's going on?

To answer that question, we must consider the prerequisite for IQ: a healthy brain. We know that good performance on one part of an IQ test, verbal reasoning, say, correlates to good performance on another feature like working memory. This is described as the 'general factor' of IQ and seems to be a feature of executive function. Executive functions are coordinated by the prefrontal cortex. So, a well-functioning PFC seems to underlie the 'general factor' of higher IQ. The highest concentration of DHA in the brain is found in the PFC.

In a 2007 analysis of ALSPAC (the study of mother and child pairs in Avon) data, Dr Joseph Hibbeln and colleagues looked at the relationship between maternal fish consumption at 32 weeks' gestation and child IQ. They found a dose-response relationship between maternal fish consumption and IQ. The more fish a mother ate during pregnancy, the higher her child's IQ. Moreover, they found no evidence of a harmful effect of high fish consumption on child health (i.e. in relation to concerns about mercury). In fact, a separate follow-up study published in 2022 found that higher maternal and umbilical cord blood levels of mercury were associated with better cognitive outcomes (higher IQ and mathematical reasoning) and no negative effects. It's not that mercury is good for the brain but that fish consumption is *so beneficial* that it cancels out potential harm from the mercury. Indeed, maternal omega-3 consumption may explicitly protect the foetus from mercury risks. This means that advice to avoid eating fish during pregnancy due to fears about mercury may have inadvertently been doing more neurological harm than good. The authors of the 2022 paper conclude that, 'Government recommendations should be reviewed to emphasise the beneficial value of fish consumption during pregnancy.' I couldn't agree more.

Brain connectivity and IQ

At the start of this book I described how we are in the habit of thinking about the mind as an ethereal, disembodied entity, rather than an emergent property of a physical brain. We make the same mistake with IQ. Challenging this idea is a recent imaging study published in 2018 which found that an individual's intelligence could be estimated from

THE PREFRONTAL CORTEX

The PFC is the area of the brain responsible for:

- Impulse control
- Delayed gratification and goal-directed behaviour
- Decision making
- Problem-solving
- Planning
- Attention
- Reasoning
- Social cognition

That is to say, many of the cognitive functions associated with intelligence and academic and social success.

patterns of their resting-state brain activity. The better the connectivity (the more connections between brain cells and how well they functioned), the higher the IQ. The participants in the study were not solving puzzles or answering any questions, they were just lying there, doing nothing. The research group used a machine learning algorithm to make the IQ predictions. To do this they input 884 brain scans and the corresponding IQ scores into the computer. This method, which the researchers themselves describe as 'coarse' and imperfect, was able to predict 20 per cent of the variance in individual intelligence from patterns of connectivity in the brain. Separate work has also shown that cortical thickness, a feature of having abundant neuronal connections, also correlates to intelligence.

As you have seen, brain connectivity is influenced by nutrition (the availability of the building blocks of brain cells), as well as cognitive challenge (learning and novelty stimulate brain cells) and stress (prolonged stress can impair brain connectivity). Cognitive ability (IQ) is one of the factors driving upward social mobility, the likelihood that a child will achieve a higher relative income or level of academic or occupational attainment than their parents.

Broadly speaking, then, being born with more connections in your brain is a good thing. Accordingly, in the previously mentioned study in mice, where they had 50 per cent fewer connections, the pups that were deprived of DHA during gestation showed deficits in a brain process called long-term potentiation (LTP). This is the method by which connections between brain cells become stronger and more likely to fire with repeated use and it is the basis of learning and memory. Insufficient DHA during pregnancy led to impaired learning in offspring. But do we see the same thing in humans?

Though deliberate restriction of an essential nutrient during pregnancy is not the kind of study that would get past a research ethics committee, it is possible to compare the outcomes for children born to mothers who had differing levels of essential fatty acid intake during pregnancy. Studies that have done this show some remarkable similarities to the animal data. For example, a study of 1,553 Dutch mother-child pairs found that maternal fatty acid status as assessed mid-pregnancy was associated with offspring grey and white matter volumes (brain cells and the connections between them): the higher the mother's blood levels of omega-3, the greater her child's brain volume at age ten.

Another research team scanned the brains of 92 one-month-old babies (born to term) and analysed the brain scan data against a range of nutrients in the mothers' diets. They found a positive correlation between the mothers' intake of omega-3 fats and the volume of the prefrontal lobes of the babies' brains. These differences were found not to be correlated with the mothers' race, education level or the household income. Actually, it's worth taking a moment to consider the characteristics of this group of mothers because they differ from the general population in a couple of key ways. First, they were highly educated: 82.65 per cent of the women had a college degree or higher, compared to 42 per cent of the general population aged over 25. And they were wealthy: 50 per cent had a household income of $100,000 or more compared to a median household income of around $67,000 for the average American, or the 30 per cent of the population who earn over $100,000. So this was a wealthy, educated group, who likely had good access to healthcare and information on staying well during pregnancy. And yet even they exhibited a variance in their intake of this essential nutrient, which correlated to alterations in their babies' brain development. What about less wealthy, less well-educated women? How do they fare in relation to this essential brain nutrient?

Data from the American National Health and Nutrition Examination Survey (NHANES) sheds some light on this question. NHANES is a national survey of the health of American citizens first conducted in 1971. It is now an annual audit, with the database providing invaluable raw data for researchers. In 2020 a study was published that looked at fatty acid status compared to ethnicity, income and education level in 44,585 people between 2003 and 2014. The results showed that, in general, fatty acid intake was low in everyone. However, it was lowest in Mexican Americans, followed by non-Hispanic white, other Hispanic, non-Hispanic Black and other (including Asian American) groups. There was also a significant interaction of education level on omega-3 intake, with those educated above high-school level consuming significantly more essential fats than those with a lower level of educational attainment. And again, those who earned more consumed more omega-3. In this group only 7.4 per cent supplemented with omega-3s; this figure was composed almost entirely of white people. That is, 6 per cent of white people were supplementing compared to less than 0.05 per cent in each of the other ethnic groups.

And us Brits?

The recommendation that UK adults should 'eat at least two portions of fish, of which one should be oily, weekly' was made in 1994. To provide some context, this was back in the days of Bill Clinton's presidency, Michael Jackson's unlikely nuptials to Elvis Presley's daughter Lisa Marie, and a young man named Jeff Bezos founding a company called Amazon. Ten years later, in 2004, the Scientific Advisory Committee on Nutrition (SACN) published a report on fish consumption.

In it they conceded that:

> *The majority of the UK population does not consume enough fish, particularly oily fish, and should be encouraged to increase consumption . . . people should eat at least two portions of fish a week, of which one should be oily. Consumption of this amount would probably confer significant public health benefits to the UK population in terms of reducing CVD [cardiovascular disease] risk. There may also be beneficial effects on foetal development . . . SACN emphasised that this recommendation represents a minimal and achievable average population goal and does not correspond to the level of fish consumption required for maximum nutritional benefit . . .*

That is, that national intake of heart-healthy oily fish was so low that getting more people to increase consumption would lead to an appreciable reduction in the number of people having heart attacks. But even this recommendation was the 'minimum'. Elsewhere in the report they also note that there is an increased demand on the mother's stores of omega-3 during pregnancy and lactation, that increased maternal intake would benefit babies, particularly those at higher risk, and that there was no evidence of adverse effects of supplementation even at high doses.

Back when UK adults were eating a third of a portion of fish per week (essentially, one generous portion per month), SACN were considering recommendations for fish consumption only in relation to its impact on heart disease and pregnancy outcomes. Not only have decades of research in the field been published since those recommendations were made – including the impact on brain development – but this period has also seen a rapid increase in the number of people reducing or eliminating animal foods from their diets. We simply do not know how many women may be consuming insufficient DHA for optimal baby brain development. My best educated guess is hardly any.

Breastfeeding

We heard earlier how breast milk is essential for the safe development of preterm babies. Breast milk is evolutionarily adapted to be the exclusive food for babies in the first months of life. Since the baby's brain is rapidly developing during this period, it should be no surprise that breast milk contains high levels of brain-essential nutrients (as well as special sugars 'designed' to feed the infant's developing gut microbiome). Breast milk contains high levels of ARA, DPA and DHA, and the DHA in formula milk does not seem to supply the brain as well as breast milk does. Correspondingly, breastfed babies have higher brain levels of DHA compared to formula-fed babies. And the levels of DHA correlate with length of breastfeeding. Of course, children who are bottle-fed thrive and reach their cognitive milestones. On an individual level differences might be hard to identify. However, when researchers look at outcomes on a population basis, children who were breastfed as babies have improved brain development, lower incidence of autism spectrum disorders and antisocial behaviours, decreased aggression and improved cognitive capacities.

But it may not be as simple as saying that 'breast is best' if we are thinking about DHA availability. A third of the DHA in breast milk is from the mother's diet. The remainder comes from the fatty acids stored in her body fat and the small amount that is produced from endogenous conversion of ALA to EPA and DHA, which is slightly higher in women than men and increases during pregnancy. The levels of DHA in breast milk will be largely dependent on those in the mother's habitual diet (or supplementation). With the currently low levels of oily fish and seafood consumption and inconsistent supplementation in the UK, it is likely to be the case that many breastfed babies are receiving below optimal levels of omega-3 fats.

So, What Should We Do?

To optimise the supply of essential fats to the rapidly developing brains of babies and infants, women should increase their consumption of oily fish (or supplements) from as early in the pregnancy as possible and through-out the duration of breastfeeding. Again, women from poorer households are disadvantaged here as seafood is more expensive per gram than indus-trially farmed poultry. A sensible intervention would be for all pregnant women to be provided with free-prescription omega-3 supplements, pro-viding 900mg per day of EPA and DHA, to ensure that no baby, irrespective of the wealth of the parents, is disadvantaged in this way.

As well as comprehensive supplementation for pregnant and breastfeeding women, I would like to see fortification in the early years, perhaps in the form of a carton of omega-3-enriched milk or low-sugar juice drink, provided to children up to the age of two. The available evidence suggests that such provision would contribute to improved behaviour, superior impulse control, lower rates of developmental dis-orders and improved cognition. Importantly, in light of the tidal wave of psychiatric diagnoses, DHA supplementation may be protective against mental illness through optimised brain development and func-tion, and enhanced stress resilience.

At the moment, in the UK, omega-3 supplements are not licensed for prescription on the NHS for anything other than to help prevent a second heart attack in those who have had one in the previous three months, or for some types of high triglycerides (fats in the blood). This conclusion is derived from data on the effects of supplementation on conditions like fatty liver and high cholesterol. But what about foetal and infant brain development? There is now an abundance of mecha-nistic-, animal- and human-imaging data to show that nutritional insufficiency of DHA has negative effects on infant brain morphology. The prevailing evidence is sufficiently robust for the European Food Safety Authority (EFSA) to deem DHA to be a 'conditionally essen-tial fatty acid for infants' and to mandate that all baby formula be fortified with it. However, there is also abundant evidence of wide-spread insufficient intake in the general population, both in relation to oily fish consumption and supplementation. Only the children of the wealthiest or most nutritionally aware (often the most wealthy) parents are likely to be getting anything close to the right amount of this essen-tial nutrient.

The emerging body of imaging data linking cortical thickness and brain connectivity to measures of intelligence should also give us pause for thought. Throughout life our brain connectivity is affected by things like the quality of our environments and the amount of stress we experience. But before we are even born, measurable differences in connectivity are influenced by the quality of maternal nutrition. If the mother's diet is deficient in key nutrients her baby's brain will not reach its full potential. Here the role of nutrition may pull together some of the controversial observations concerning class and IQ, that the corn-flakes at the top just inherited 'better genes'. We have seen how higher income and educational attainment mean that a woman is more likely to consume greater levels of DHA, helping to lay down more robust foundations in her baby's brain. In this way, the children of wealthy, educated mothers don't just enter the world with a sociological advan-tage, they have a neurological one too.

There is a risk that in highlighting the crucial role of maternal health and nutrition on her infant's brain development and future mental health I am accused of 'blaming' mothers, of heaping on the guilt. As if the physical burden and identity transformation weren't enough, should mothers feel totally responsible for all future psycho-logical difference or distress that their children develop too? No. My case is not one of blame. Most mothers I have met and worked with blame themselves enough to begin with, even when they know they have tried their very best. Rather, in pointing out the essential nature of the health of the mother I hope to support the case for better infor-mation and support for women preconception, during pregnancy and after birth. Such support cannot come only in the form of nutrition – since this is just one of the elements provided by the maternal universe. But it is a start.

In summary, population intake of brain-building essential fatty acids is low in both UK and US populations. Animal studies and cor-relational human data indicate that these low levels of omega-3 intake during pregnancy have detrimental effects on brain development, including inhibited growth of brain cells, poorer neuronal communica-tion, reduced brain connectivity and smaller regional and overall brain volumes. Further to this, the burden of this nutritional insufficiency falls predominantly on poor people and ethnic minorities. By virtue of being born to poor parents or as a member of a marginalised group, these children start their lives at a neurological disadvantage, the effects of which compound over time.

We have spent some time thinking about the irreplaceable role of DHA on baby's brain development, but what about other nutrients?

CHAPTER 5

CHOLINE – THE GAME-CHANGING NUMBER TWO

I'M AWARE I have spent a lot of time explaining why DHA is so important for brain health. But evidence is emerging that DHA falls short of its potential without the support of choline. If DHA is one of the building blocks of brain cells, then choline is the mortar; and just as necessary for building strong neurological foundations. You may not have heard much about choline but I hope that by the end of this chapter you will have a newfound appreciation for this unsung nutritional hero.

Choline is a nutrient that is 'conditionally essential' during pregnancy, considered critical for normal brain development. However, research establishes that it remains important throughout lactation, weaning and early childhood. So what does it do?

- **Acetylcholine** – Acetylcholine is an important neurotransmitter. Not only is it essential for the function of muscles, but it is the major neurotransmitter of the parasympathetic nervous system (aka the 'rest and digest' system and the opposite of the 'fight or flight' response). Within the brain, acetylcholine plays a key role in cognitive function, memory and learning. Low intake of choline is associated with decreased levels of acetylcholine in the brain.

- **Cell membranes** – You know by now that cell membranes are largely composed of fats, an important constituent of which is DHA. However, DHA is not the only fat in town. A raft of choline derivatives are also crucial for the formation and integrity of all cell membranes.

- **Myelin** – Myelin is a fatty substance that insulates the axon of a nerve. It helps to accelerate the speed of action potentials, the rate at which a nerve sends a signal. It is the myelin that becomes irreparably damaged in neurodegenerative diseases such as multiple sclerosis. The metabolites of choline are essential for repairing damaged myelin.

- **Homocysteine** – Homocysteine is an amino acid, high levels of which are a marker of increased risk of neural tube defects, stroke, schizophrenia and depression. Homocysteine can be converted to the (non-harmful) essential amino acid methionine by two biological pathways. One pathway depends on B vitamins (B6, B9 and B12). You will see later in the chapter on the aging brain the powerful effect of vitamin B supplementation on homocysteine and neurodegeneration. The other pathway requires a choline derivative, making choline important for protecting your body from the harmful effects of high homocysteine. In turn, methionine is a precursor for one of the body's most important antioxidants (glutathione), protecting the body from the harmful effects of reactive oxygen species, which can damage DNA.

- **Gene expression** – The behaviour of your cells is not simply about whether you have the gene or not, but whether (and in some cases, to what degree) it is active. A range of environmental stimuli can influence whether a gene will be turned on or not (aka silenced). Nutritional status is also a potent modulator of gene expression. While we interact with the environment through all of our senses, the act of eating is a primary means by which we *take the environment in*. For this reason, the quality of a person's nutrition is a powerful piece of information for their genes about the conditions of their environment. Choline deficiency during pregnancy alters the DNA of brain cells and reduces the rate of neurogenesis.

Effects of Choline Deficiency During Pregnancy

During pregnancy a very large amount of choline is delivered to the baby, indicating that it plays a crucially important role in foetal development (biomagnification in action again!). In animal studies supplemental choline improves the formation of blood vessels in the placenta and the quality of placental blood flow, vital for the supply of nutrients to the developing foetus.

But we have a problem. The choline adequate intake (AI) for pregnant women in the US (450mg per day) is based on the amount for non-pregnant women plus 25mg, which itself is extrapolated from just one study . . . conducted on men. This means that there has been no formal investigation as to how much choline women should be consuming to ensure that there is sufficient supply for the baby's developing brain.

One illuminating paper from the US highlights the urgent need for more evidence. In this study women were randomised to two groups of choline supplementation during the third trimester of pregnancy. One group received a supplement of the recommended adequate intake of choline. The second group received nearly double that amount, 930mg per day. Seven years later the researchers revisited the families and assessed the children on tests of attention. The children participated in a very repetitive, very boring computer-based task in which they had to press a button to indicate whether they had seen a low-contrast grey square on a pale grey background. This version of the sustained attention task (SAT) has 216 rounds. Without any other stimuli (such as colours or sound effects) to keep them engaged, the SAT is a very good indicator of a child's ability to focus and pay attention. When they compared performance, the children of the mothers who received the higher dose of choline were better able to sustain attention and were more accurate in their responses – they provided fewer false positives. Though this was a small trial of just 20 children, it is consistent with other trials and with the animal data: increased maternal choline intake during pregnancy is associated with long-term improved cognition in children.

Of course, the ability to pay attention goes further than being able to perform well in boring laboratory tasks. Simply put, children who can pay attention do better in school. The ability to pay attention is a predictor of school grades in literacy, vocabulary and maths above the contribution of IQ. That is, school performance seems to be less about being naturally gifted and more about how well you can stay focused on the problem at hand.

Furthermore, it indicates that the current AI recommendations might well be far from adequate for the needs of pregnant women. For those of us in the UK and Europe, currently the European Food Safety Authority recommends 480mg and 520mg per day of choline for pregnant and lactating women respectively. Half the amount shown to be beneficial in recent studies. Of additional concern is that an analysis of dietary intake indicates that typical choline consumption in adults is below the recommended levels, at 291–468mg per day.

Food Sources of Choline

Unsurprisingly, given its role in cell membrane formation and neuro-transmitter synthesis, a woman's stores of choline are depleted during pregnancy when her body is building her baby's big, hungry brain. She must keep her levels topped up through what she eats. On the next page is a graph of the best food sources of choline.

Women are advised to avoid liver and liver products (such as liver pâté and liver sausage) during pregnancy as it is a rich source of vitamin A in retinol form. Though vitamin A is an important nutrient for health and development, in high doses, especially early in pregnancy, it can cause foetal malformations, particularly in the head, face and brain. Beta-carotene (from plants) that the body then converts into vitamin A does not have these effects. Consequently, eggs are the next best food source of choline during pregnancy.

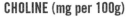

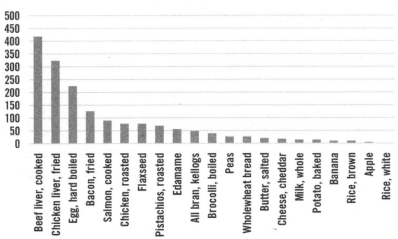

CHOLINE (mg per 100g)

US national health survey data indicates that it is difficult for most adults to achieve sufficient choline intake without the consumption of eggs or a supplement. At this time, comparative data is not available for the UK. However, a British Vegan Society survey found that during the coronavirus pandemic 12.3 per cent of people had cut back on the consumption of eggs and dairy.

Choline and DHA: The Dream Team

We often talk about nutrients as if they work alone. Vitamin C is important for wound healing. Vitamin A is good for your eyes. In reality, nutrients are not solo entrepreneurs. They are collaborators, working together to support each other's biological pathways and the overall health of the organism (that is to say, you). A recent clinical study demonstrated the partnership between choline and DHA in a way that has important implications not just for the developing brain but also for the aging brain and neurodegeneration.

A randomised controlled trial (RCT) in which 30 pregnant women were split into two groups and provided with the following from about

12 weeks' gestation to delivery:

1. 500mg choline + 50mg labelled choline* + 200mg DHA + pregnancy vitamins
2. 25mg labelled choline* + 200mg DHA + pregnancy vitamins

   *Labelling the choline allowed the researchers to track its activity in the body.

They found that adding choline increased availability of DHA. So choline helps the body and brain to take up the DHA that we all know, love and need more of. This study raises an important concern. Only 10 per cent of the US adult population and only 8 per cent of pregnant women are consuming the AI of choline (remembering that this may be too low anyway). What impact is this having on cognitive function at a population level? Given the established link between maternal choline and offspring attention, could this explain the rapid rise in disorders of inattention over recent decades?

I spoke to Kevin Klatt PhD, a registered dietitian, nutrition researcher and lead author on the choline supplementation in pregnancy study described above. I asked him how we come to pregnancy nutrition recommendations:

Oh man! This taps into how do we even know what non-pregnant people need? Because, often, recommendations are taking the non-pregnant recommendation value and modifying it. You've opened a Pandora's box with that question!

I say we start with animal models, but in many ways, you often rely then on [human] observational data, which is what led us to the folic acid–neural tube defect link that you would've never really uncovered by animal models. And so it is in some ways a serendipitous thing, which is also a bias thing. And I would say that I can point you to different nutrients where our emphasis on that comes from these primate models or these rodent models or human epidemiology. When you dig deep into the data for dietary recommendations for pregnancy it's assumptions upon assumptions upon assumptions and that there's almost no experimental data. And that's pretty con-cerning in many ways . . . Often what's been done is just this sort of mass balance approach where you're [saying]: 'Assuming only a structural role of choline in membranes, how much choline would you need to support the development of the placenta and everything in the foetal compartment?' But there's many assumptions that go into that line of thinking and it really doesn't have any experimen-tal evidence to support that higher than that isn't better.

The Choline Science Summit is a scientific meeting where experts in the field of choline research meet to discuss findings, implications and calls to action in light of the best available evidence of the role of choline on health. One of the recommendations of the 2018 meeting was that 'choline must be integrated into the prenatal supplement regimen'. At the time of writing that was four years ago, so I thought I would check out the choline status of pregnancy vitamins in the UK. My findings are presented below:

Product	Choline (mg per recommended serving)
Active Iron Pregnancy Plus	0
Bassetts Vitamins During Pregnancy Strawberry & Orange Flavour Pastilles	0
Boots Breastfeeding Essential Vitamins + Omega-3	0
Boots Pregnancy Essential Vitamins	0
Proceive Advanced Fertility Supplement Max Women	0
Proceive Pregnancy Supplement Trimester 1	40 (as choline bitartrate)
Proceive Pregnancy Supplement Trimester 2	0
Proceive Pregnancy Supplement Trimester 3	0
Seven Seas Pregnancy Plus Breastfeeding Vitamins	0
Seven Seas Pregnancy Vitamins with Folic Acid	0
Viridian Pregnancy Complex	50 (as choline bitartrate)
Vitabiotics Pregnacare Original	0

(Continued on the next page)

Product	Choline (mg per recommended serving)
Vitabiotics Pregnacare Max	0
Vitabiotics Pregnacare Plus Omega-3	0
Vitabiotics Pregnacare Before Conception	0

Despite being essential for healthy brain development during pregnancy and early childhood, and recommended by the world's leading scientists, hardly any UK pregnancy supplements contain choline. The ones that do contain it don't do so in anything near sufficient amounts. This would not be a problem if it was established that there was adequate intake in the general population from habitual diet; however, this is not the case. Most people are not eating enough. Furthermore, pregnancy and lactation increase the demand for choline. If this demand is not met then what we face is generation after generation of declining choline status, which may manifest in autism and problems with memory. Low levels in the population and a lack of guidance from government is compromising the optimal brain development of generations of babies born in the UK and US, and perhaps beyond. Our governments must act urgently to establish RDAs (recommended daily amounts) for choline, improve professional education on the importance of this nutrient and institute a programme of public health information, especially for pregnant and lactating women, and young children.

Such strong scientific endorsement for a nutrient that is key to infant brain development sounds like a huge selling point for a pregnancy supplement. So, why isn't it added? The answer is convenience. Choline salts are rather bulky; they don't compact down into one easy-to-swallow pill, especially not alongside all the other nutrients in a pregnancy supplement. Supplement companies would have to reformulate their products, perhaps incurring additional production and packaging costs, which would cut into profits. There is also no demand from the consumer for a supplement containing choline (because nobody knows). However, I think if people were made aware of its function and the high rates of insufficiency, the idea of taking the sup-plements might be an easier pill to swallow.

Choline and Autism – Is There a Link?

I hesitated to write this section for several reasons. The first is that the increasing rates of diagnosis have led to a lot of harmful misinforma-tion as to the causes of autism. Misinformation only delays people accessing the right support and treatment. Another reason is that for those who consider autism and autistic behavioural traits to be a vari-ation of human neurology (termed neurodivergence) the suggestion that some cases might be prevented may be considered insulting. From the position of neurodivergence, autism is a difference (like colour blindness) or a disability, depending on the severity. Not a disease to be cured. However, the scientific consensus is that autism is a neurodevel-opmental disorder, with late pregnancy (after 22 weeks) identified as a critical period for its development.

While I am certain that many, perhaps the majority of, autism cases arise spontaneously, there is a growing body of research literature on the in utero conditions that are associated with an increased incidence of autism. For example, prenatal maternal stress is a significant predic-tor of autistic traits, especially in males. A meta-analysis published in 2021 showed an association between maternal infection or fever dur-ing pregnancy and increased risk of autism. The researchers estimate that incidence of autism would drop by 12–17 per cent if infection during pregnancy could be prevented. Maternal autoantibody-related autism spectrum disorder involves harmful antibodies from the mother's immune system crossing the placenta, entering the foetal brain and causing alterations in neural development. When the mother's blood during pregnancy contains these antibodies there is an eight times increased risk that the child will have autism.

These studies highlight the fact that *in utero* exposures have a bearing on the likelihood of a child developing autism. There is con-verging evidence for the availability of choline as a risk factor of autism.

One study compared brain tissue samples of deceased individuals, looking at the hallmarks of cholinergic activity in the brains of autistic people, people with non-autistic neurodevelopmental impairment, and healthy controls. It found that a cholinergic receptor called M_1 was significantly lower (up to 30 per cent) in people with autism compared to the other two groups.

Many autistic people experience difficulties associated with sensory processing, such as a heightened sensitivity to sudden or loud noises. This processing of sensory information depends on the action of acetylcholine. A recent paper used computer modelling to investigate the potential of nutritional choline to improve sensory processing in autism. To do this, the research team collated the data on two sets of genes: those that are associated with autistic spectrum disorders and those involved in cholinergic signalling. They found several points of interaction for both choline and acetylcholine and conclude that dietary choline is a low-risk intervention for cell signalling and the availability of acetylcholine in autistic people.

Finally, a systematic review of the use of Alzheimer's disease medications to treat autism found improvements in 'expressive language and communication, receptive language, social interaction, irritability, hyperactivity, attention, eye contact, emotional lability, repetitive or self-stimulatory behaviors, motor planning, disruptive behaviors, obsessive-compulsive symptoms, lethargy, overall ASD behaviors, and increased REM sleep'. Of significance is that these drugs work by increasing the availability of acetylcholine, either by preventing it from being broken down or by stimulating its increased release.

While none of these studies is conclusive by itself, it seems to me that the patterns of response to choline treatment provide grounds for further research on levels of maternal choline intake and autism risk, and the use of supplemental choline as a means to modify symptoms.

If a relationship is identified between maternal choline and offspring autism it should be made clear that the mothers should not carry the burden of responsibility. You can only act on the information that you have and, as described, despite scientists knowing that choline is essential for healthy brain development, neither the UK nor US governments, nor the EFSA, have established recommended daily amounts of the nutrient in pregnancy. Furthermore, many healthcare professionals are not aware of the importance of choline and it is the least likely of the common nutrients to be recommended to patients as part of a healthy diet. This shows us that there is a lot of work to do; before we can educate the public, we have to educate the professionals. Our governments should act urgently to answer these research questions and, where necessary, provide clear advice and information to the public.

Should choline be able to mitigate some of the symptoms of autism, not only would this offer some relief to many thousands of individuals and their families, but it could do so with minimal side effects. Both dietary and supplemental choline are well tolerated and do not interfere with medication.

TAKE ACTION

As I have shown, omega-3s and choline are essential for brain development. It is also evident that population intakes of these nutrients are low, weakening the very foundations of brain health from conception.

Ask the good people at the National Institute for Health and Care Excellence (NICE) why, given the established importance of choline for brain development, the nutrient is not included in pregnancy nutrition guidelines. You can contact them at https://www.nice.org.uk/get-involved/contact-us

---

As things currently stand, in women of childbearing age:

- 90 per cent have an inadequate intake of choline.
- 88 per cent have insufficient levels of folate.
- 67 per cent are iodine-deficient.
- An average of just 8.6g of oily fish per day is consumed, around a third of the minimum recommended intake.

There has been some movement towards improving the diets of British mothers. Pregnant women in the poorest households are eligible for the government's Healthy Start vouchers – a prepaid card providing £4.25 per week to purchase plain cow's milk; fresh, frozen or tinned fruits; vegetables; grains and pulses; infant formula; and vitamins.

However, awareness and uptake of the programme is poor, with up to 50 per cent of eligible women in some areas not receiving the benefit. Furthermore, not all households on low incomes qualify, only those earning less than £408 per month after tax. This leaves hundreds of thousands of households missing out on valuable pregnancy nutrition.

A TALE OF TWO BRAINS

Anya and Mia were born at exactly the same time, 2.16pm on a warm June afternoon in a north London hospital. Their mothers, Yasmin and Zoe, smiled weakly at one another from their neighbouring beds on the busy maternity ward. Anya was born two days after her due date, weighing in at 7lb 2oz. Mia was a little early, born at 36 weeks and three days and weighing 6lb 8oz. Both baby girls were pronounced healthy and well by the doctor.

Yasmin took Anya home. Her mother was overjoyed to meet her granddaughter. She had stocked Yasmin's freezer with home-cooked meals that she could easily reheat. Yasmin breastfed Anya for six months before introducing weaning foods. She started with homemade rice porridge (overcooked rice mixed with a little breast milk), gradually adding other foods to it like mashed banana, puréed sweet potato and spinach. This was a good intuitive strategy as research indicates that introducing vegetables with baby rice increases baby's acceptance of them, making it easier to incorporate them into the daily diet later. Baby Anya also developed a taste for bread crusts and hard-boiled egg yolks.

Mia was a hungry baby whose breast milk was supplemented with formula. Zoe checked with the health visitor to make sure she bought the best one. Due to the biomagnification of key nutrients, breastfed babies have a higher intake of brain-supportive essential fats and choline than formula-fed infants. Like her mother, Mia was weaned on packaged baby rice (finely milled rice, mixed with milk) and Farley's Rusks (biscuits designed as a weaning food for babies). Zoe was pleased to see that both came with added vitamins. Mia liked mashed potato and the ready-made baby-food meal pouches but it was harder to get her to eat anything with 'green' in it. The added sugars in the pre-packed baby biscuits (with 4.9g in every biscuit, they are nearly a third sugar) will begin to shape baby Mia's taste preferences for sweeter foods (more on this later). Similarly, the smooth, uniform texture and appearance of pre-packaged baby food can make it more difficult for children to accept the taste and textures of home-cooked and less-processed foods.

Part III

DISREPAIR – HOW MODERN DIETS HARM BRAIN HEALTH IN CHILDHOOD, ADOLESCENCE AND YOUNG ADULTHOOD

CHAPTER 6

SUGAR

I KNOW, I know. You can't open a news article nowadays without someone shouting at you about how sugar is the cause of all your problems, from acne to constipation. But I reckon you have heard less about the relationship between sugar and the brain. And it might surprise you to know that it's not all bad news. Believe me, as a keen baker with a penchant for jam-making, I'm not here to ban sugar completely. I mean, there is some bad news but I hope to provide you with a nuanced take on what sugar is doing to your brain and mental health. So let's talk.

First, a question. Do you have a sweet tooth? Whether you prefer cheese over chocolate, if you are human then technically the answer to this question is yes. Humans have an inbuilt liking for sugar for reasons that are very cool for a food nerd like me.

Glucose – What, How and Why?

Glucose is a simple sugar and the preferred energy source for almost all the cells in your body, including your brain. It is predominantly synthesised by plants as a product of photosynthesis. Plants concentrate their glucose into fruits to make them enticing to herbivorous and omnivorous animals and humans. When fruits and berries are consumed so are their seeds (think about the seeds on a strawberry or within a fig). The eater wanders off, the seeds survive digestion and are deposited in a new location in a near-perfect growing medium (faeces). In this way, humans and animals are in a mutually profitable relationship with plants: they provide a concentrated source of energy and we help with seed dispersal. It's the same deal that bees have with flowers: nectar in exchange for pollination. Coevolution is cool.

For this reason, almost all naturally sweet foods – fruit, tubers, honey, etc. – are safe to eat, and sweet flavours elicit a reward response in the brain to encourage us to return to this valuable fuel source. All plants produce sucrose, a molecule of glucose bound to a molecule of fructose. This is processed and refined to produce table sugar.

Strictly, glucose is not just the brain's preferred energy source, but its absolutely essential one. Even if someone were to eliminate all carbohydrates and free sugars from the diet, their body would convert protein into glucose through a process called gluconeogenesis to supply the brain. If they were not eating enough protein then the body would start to break down their own muscles to generate glucose. Your brain prefers glucose to fat specifically because of the way that your cells convert fat and glucose into the body's units of energy called adenosine triphosphate (ATP). Converting fat into ATP requires more oxygen compared to glucose. This means that the brain would run out of oxygen more quickly running on fat, which is something, of course, we would like to avoid.

The second reason relates to oxidation. As I mentioned earlier (see chapter 2) the fats that are essential for the maintenance of a healthy brain are very unsaturated, which makes them prone to oxidation. Oxidative damage hurts the brain. Using fat for energy produces more superoxide (a major reactive oxygen species), which would risk causing damage to brain cells.

So glucose it is! The body is able to extract all the glucose that it needs from wholegrains and starchy vegetables. This means that, strictly, only people undertaking intense or prolonged exercise likely need to consume a pure source of glucose. In reality, though, the supply of glucose in the Western diet is very high due to the presence of free and added sugars in processed foods. 'Added sugars' are refined sugars used in food preparation and as table sugar. 'Free sugars' include 'added sugars' plus those naturally present in honey and syrups, as well as in fruit and vegetable juices and juice concentrates.

Types of Sugar

If you see any of the below on your list of ingredients, that food contains sugar. In addition, 'concentrated apple juice' and 'concentrated grape juice' are just ways for food manufacturers to get away with saying no added (table) sugar. But if you boil away the water from grape or apple juice you are left with a sticky, sweet glucose-fructose syrup. It's sugar. Don't let them fool you.

- Agave syrup/nectar
- Brown rice syrup/rice syrup
- Coconut sugar
- Corn syrup
- Date syrup
- Dextrose
- Fructose
- Glucose
- High-fructose corn syrup
- Honey
- Icing sugar/powdered sugar/confectioner's sugar
- Invert sugar syrup/invert sugar
- Lactose
- Light and dark brown sugar
- Malt syrup
- Maltose
- Maple syrup
- Molasses
- Muscovado sugar
- Table sugar/white sugar/granulated sugar/caster sugar/sucrose

SUGAR: HOW MUCH IS TOO MUCH?

The UK government recommends that free sugars – sugars added to food or drinks, and sugars found naturally in honey, syrups and unsweetened fruit and vegetable juices, smoothies and purées – should not make up more than 5 per cent of the energy (calories) you get from food and drink each day.

This means:

- Children aged 4–6 should have no more than 19g of free sugars a day (five sugar cubes).
- Children aged 7–10 should have no more than 24g of free sugars a day (six sugar cubes).
- Adults should have no more than 30g of free sugars a day (roughly equivalent to seven sugar cubes).

There is currently no guideline limit for children under the age of four (who knows why), but it is recommended they avoid sugar-sweetened drinks and food with sugar added to it. In the US experts recommend that children under the age of two do not consume *any* foods with free sugars. This includes the usual suspects chocolate, cakes, biscuits, ice cream. However, many 'wholesome' foods promoted as good meal and snack choices for kids, such as granola and fruity snack bars, yoghurts, juices and juice drinks, can have high levels of sugar.

In order to know whether a food is considered high or low in sugar, you have to turn over the packet and scan the nutritional information. Look for the column that reads 'per 100g'.

- High: more than 22.5g of total sugars per 100g
- Low: 5g or less of total sugars per 100g

If the brain needs glucose so badly, why is too much sugar a bad thing? The neurological consequences of diabetes can help us to answer this question.

Insulin Resistance and Diabetes

Diabetes mellitus is a health condition characterised by long-term elevated blood glucose. When you eat starchy or sugary foods, enzymes in your mouth and stomach start to break apart the larger molecules into their constituent subunits. The liberated glucose is absorbed in your small intestine and crosses into the bloodstream, causing your blood sugar (glucose) levels to rise. Some of this glucose will be absorbed into muscles, especially if you have been recently active, but if sugar hangs around in the blood too long it can trigger a range of health complications that I will describe in a moment.

The removal of excess glucose from the blood is the main job of insulin, a hormone secreted by the pancreas. When receptors on the surface of a cell detect insulin, it activates glucose transporters to pull glucose from the blood into the cell, where it can be used for respiration or stored in muscles or fat. In general terms diabetes is the failure or insufficiency of this process.

There are two main types of diabetes: type 1 and type 2. Type 1 diabetes mellitus (T1DM) is an autoimmune condition. The body's immune cells attack the beta cells in the pancreas that produce insulin so insufficient insulin is produced. Type 2 diabetes mellitus (T2DM) is typically associated with diet and lifestyle factors such as adiposity and physical inactivity. Over 90 per cent of diabetes cases in the UK are type 2. Here, cells become *insensitive* to insulin. It's like when you live near a busy road; initially you might find yourself responding to every passing car, but over time it becomes background noise that you no longer notice.

Insulin moves glucose into cells and storage but this is not its only job. Insulin, and two similar compounds helpfully named insulin-like growth factor 1 and 2, are *neurotrophic factors*, they support the survival of neurones. So when brain cells become insensitive to insulin, not only do they experience a reduction in energy availability, but they lose the protection of these growth factors.

So having too much sugar in your blood over a long period of time can overwhelm your body's ability to process it, and throw your body out of balance. What happens then?

Hyperglycaemia (high blood sugar) disturbs the function of the endothelial cells that line blood vessels, causing damage. Remembering that your very active, very hungry brain is fed by hundreds of miles of veins and capillaries, damage to these blood vessels cuts off the supply of nutrients and oxygen to brain cells. But it gets worse. Damage to blood vessels increases oxidative stress, the damage caused by an excess of reactive oxygen species. Oxidative stress has been conclusively shown to be an independent driver of Alzheimer's disease. So now we have damaged blood vessels and brain cells that are both starved of oxygen and nutrients as well as suffering oxidative damage. But it gets worse.

High blood sugar also impairs a process called autophagy, which you can think of as the brain's garbage disposal. Autophagy helps to get rid of worn-out mitochondria (the powerhouse of the cell) and cellular waste. If these are not cleared away, they can further increase the oxidative stress burden. High sugar intake also lowers circulating levels of brain-derived neurotrophic factor (BDNF), the compound required for the protection of nerves.

So, now we have a situation where brain cells are starved of nutrients and oxygen, burdened with toxic waste *and* deprived of crucial repair mechanisms. In this way long-term elevated blood glucose is an all-out assault on your nerves.

Given all that, it makes sense that one of the common complications of diabetes is nerve damage. In fact, *up to 50 per cent* of people with diabetes experience some form of mild or moderate neuropathy:

- **Sensory** – Damage to sensory nerves that detect temperature and touch/pressure.

- **Motor neuropathy** – Damage to nerves responsible for movement.
- **Autonomic** – Damage affecting non-voluntary actions like heartbeat.

The most obvious of these is sensory neuropathy. The function of pain is as a warning signal, informing you of the risk or presence of tissue damage. If your nerves are not functioning properly, you could hurt yourself and not realise. Damaged tissue that is not treated can soon become infected (high blood sugar also slows wound healing), and if the subsequent infection is not treated the damage can be irreparable. A report from the Food Foundation, published in 2022, showed that diabetes-related amputations had increased by 23 per cent in the previous five years. It is a similar story elsewhere. After years of decline, diabetic amputations rose by 50 per cent in the USA, driven by sharp increases in young and middle-aged people requiring surgery.

While damage to the sensory nerves of the hands and feet is easy to recognise, what is less obvious, until it is too late, is the damage to brain cells. If neurones die within your brain you will not know until the damage creates symptoms such as forgetfulness or changes in mood. And indeed this is what we see.

Diabetes and Dementia Risk

The relationship between T2DM and dementia is well established. Diabetes increases the risk of mild cognitive impairment, vascular dementia and Alzheimer's disease, and the longer someone has diabetes (and prediabetes) the higher the risk. We should be concerned about this relationship between diabetes duration and increased dementia because growing numbers of children around the world are being diagnosed with type 2 diabetes. Children who develop T2DM will live with the condition for decades. What impact will this have on their long-term brain health, and the mental health of an entire future generation? Will the nation be able to care for them?

An American study published in 2022 showed that there had been an increase in new cases of T2DM in children and adolescents during the Covid-19 pandemic, especially in those from poorer households. A study in India found a similar result in adults, linking the increased risk to the weight that many people gained during lockdown when movement was restricted and one of the few pleasures left to many was food.

Elevated blood sugar, prediabetes and T2DM confer significant risks of cognitive decline and neurodegeneration. The longer someone lives with these conditions, the greater the brain harm. Dementia is already our leading cause of death. We can only expect rates to dramatically increase if we do nothing to improve population glucose management.

THIAMINE

Elevated blood sugar (as seen in type 1 and type 2 diabetes) is associated with significantly reduced levels of thiamine (vitamin B1). It seems that the kidneys of people with diabetes excrete very high levels of thiamine in urine. Thiamine is essential for healthy nerves and a deficiency can cause cognitive impairments including confusion and memory deficits (see page 93).

Gestational Diabetes

During pregnancy it is normal and natural for a woman's insulin levels to increase. This is an evolutionary mechanism that allows her body to prepare for the energetic demands of late-stage pregnancy and breastfeeding by increasing fat storage. However, if levels drift too far upwards, she may be diagnosed with gestational diabetes. A body mass index (BMI) above 30 is the main modifiable risk factor for gestational diabetes. Other risk factors include higher maternal age and a family history of diabetes.

Gestational diabetes increases the risk of serious birth complications like pre-eclampsia (dangerously high blood pressure and organ damage) and depression. Babies born to diabetic mothers are at increased risk of developing a condition called macrosomia, which means they are very big. This can make vaginal birth more dangerous, sometimes impossible. As a safety measure these babies are delivered early, often by Caesarean section. I described earlier the brain health risk associated with preterm delivery. These babies are also more likely to be born with low blood sugar. These complications might explain why children born to diabetic mothers seem to have poorer cognitive outcomes compared to children born to mothers with normal blood glucose. Babies born to mothers with gestational diabetes have an increased risk of developing type 2 diabetes when they grow up, with the brain health risks that come with that.

A meta-analysis that included data of over 6,000 children found that infants of diabetic mothers had poorer cognitive development scores, and indications of poorer IQ (too few studies measured IQ for them to be sure). Other work, though, has shown a greater risk of cognitive impairment in children of diabetic mothers. A longitudinal study that looked at children's academic outcomes concluded that children of mothers with gestational diabetes had significantly lower IQs compared to the children of women without the condition. Gestational diabetes impairs the transfer of DHA from mother to foetus, which is likely to be one of the key mechanisms underlying the cognitive deficit seen in children of diabetic mothers.

The good news is that we can reduce these risks for mother and baby. In a study published in 2019, five UK maternity units randomised women with diabetes risk factors to either a Mediterranean-style (minimally processed) diet or their usual intake. The characteristics of the trial diet were a 'high intake of nuts [30g per day], extra virgin olive oil [500ml per week], fruit, vegetables, non-refined grains, and legumes; moderate to high consumption of fish; low to moderate intake of poultry and dairy products such as yoghurt and cheese; low consumption of red meat and processed meat; and avoidance of sugary drinks, fast food and food rich in animal fat'. Women on the Mediterranean diet had a 35 per cent reduced risk of developing gestational diabetes.

Sugar and Stress

Chocolate. Ice cream. A lovely slice of cake. Have you ever wondered why so many of our favourite comfort foods are sweet? There is a regulatory relationship between the major stress hormone, cortisol, and sugar. Cortisol is a glucocorticoid and the clue is in the prefix 'gluco' – one of cortisol's main jobs is to ensure, when you are in a state of potential threat or danger, that there is enough glucose available to both fuel your muscles and feed your brain as it works out the best way to help you escape the danger or manage the threat. And this relationship works in both directions; sugar consumption has been shown to blunt the rise of cortisol in response to psychological stress. So stress and blood sugar go hand in hand.

People who live in poverty or who have lower social status, particularly in highly unequal societies like the UK and US, have an increased risk of developing type 2 diabetes and the associated health complications. In part this is because, as we will see in the next chapter, the food that is affordable on lower incomes tends to be more refined, lower in fibre and higher in free and added sugars. However, the stress of poverty and inequality *itself* can create changes in the body that increase risk.

Human beings do not have protective shells like turtles. We do not have the porcupine's prickly spines or the viper's venom. When we experience existential or psychological threat our best chances of survival are our accumulated resources. If we are lucky, that means a good social support network and some financial savings. Our main *internal* resource is energy. In the long term that means a ready supply of fat to help us survive the 'lean times'. In the short term that means elevated blood glucose to fuel our brain and muscles.

A scientific literature review published in 2020 showed that cortisol is typically elevated in people who have chronically low social status. This group also show poorer recovery from acute stress; that is, it takes them longer to return to their already elevated baseline than someone with higher social status. Essentially, being poor or of lower social status is perceived by the brain as a threat, a stress, and cortisol rises to provide the brain-body with energy to manage the threat. When cortisol rises, more sugar is released from the liver. Cortisol also turns on a gene that promotes the formation of glucose from sources like pyruvate and lactate. This is the stress response in action. The problem is that the stress response is not adapted to be elevated over long periods of time. The changes that occur in the body that are adaptive for acute stress (such as increased blood sugar and fat and increased blood pressure) become harmful over the long term and predispose low-status individuals to metabolic health issues. This process is called 'stress-induced hyperglycaemia'. This makes addressing social inequality one of the most important but unaddressed public health interventions. Unbelievably, despite the most recent Office for National Statistics data showing that the UK has seen 'statistically significant increases in the inequality in life expectancy at birth since 2015', plans for a white paper designed to address health inequality were reportedly scrapped by former health secretary Thérèse Coffey.

One of the other negative consequences of prolonged stress is the inhibition of the hormone leptin. Food intake is an intricate and complex process that depends on the balance between hormones that initiate eating and those that turn it off. Leptin is one of the key satiety hormones and it is produced by fat cells and specialised cells in the small intestine. Levels of leptin rise after a meal or as we start to increase our fat stores. Essentially, it is a signal to the brain that 'we have enough energy on board, we can stop eating now, thanks'. So far, so good.

Typically, insulin increases leptin, which makes sense, right? Insulin is released in response to a rise in blood glucose, which indicates that we have just eaten, so we turn off hunger. However, long-term high insulin, as seen in diabetes or stress-induced hyperglycaemia, can promote leptin resistance. The result is that a brain-body that is in a state of prolonged stress thinks that it is starving. This nudges the person into a vicious cycle in which they are stressed but they are not responding to leptin so feel hungry; they crave carbohydrate-rich foods (to provide energy and switch off cortisol) but these foods push up blood glucose and insulin. Stress also promotes the release of inflammatory cytokines, immune signalling molecules, which, over the long term, can damage tissues, including neurones, and interfere with the production of neurotransmitters. These and other factors lead to a deterioration in physical and mental health.

There is perhaps no starker example of this than the huge difference in healthy life expectancy in the UK, where the most deprived women and men can, respectively, expect 19.3 and 18.6 fewer years of healthy life than the wealthiest.

Sugar-Sweetened Beverages

So far, I have been talking about the sugar found in food. However, liquid sugars, found in sugar-sweetened beverages (SSBs), deserve some consideration because, compared to sugars found in food, they seem to have a separate and unique negative impact on immune activity and brain health.

In an analysis of 1,234 mother-child pairs, published in 2018, there was an inverse correlation between maternal SSB consumption and child IQ as measured at ages three and seven. For every additional daily serving of SSBs, child IQ was between 1.2 and 1.7 points lower in mid-childhood. Consumption of SSBs in early childhood was linked to 2.4 fewer IQ points per single daily serving. Curiously, switching to diet soda did not help, an inverse association remained. Similarly, another study found that the children of mothers who drank more SSBs during breastfeeding had poorer cognitive outcomes at the age of two. The research team highlighted that it was the fructose (in drinks not whole fruit) content of these beverages that correlated with poorer cognition. When a mother consumes SSBs, the fructose concentration in her breast milk increases. Since newborns feed every couple of hours, this means frequent exposure to fructose.

OMEGA-3 AND DIABETES

A small study of older people published in 2008 found that a diet high in omega-3 (720g of oily fish per week plus 15ml of sardine oil daily) increased insulin sensitivity and reduced markers of

---

inflammation. A larger study published in 2013 found the same thing. Here, people with overweight and type 2 diabetes took either 2g of omega-3 EPA for 12 weeks or a corn oil placebo. After three months the EPA group had significantly lower HbA1c, a marker of long-term blood glucose and reduced insulin. More recently, in 2018, a meta-analysis of 45 randomised controlled trials involving 2,674 people confirmed the finding: increased omega-3 intake improved blood fats, reduced inflammation and improved insulin sensitivity. These findings offer potential treatment options for patients alongside lifestyle modification, or for those who take metformin and suffer side effects (nausea, vomiting, diarrhoea) that make the medication difficult to tolerate.

It also raises the question (for researchers) whether, as well as the high levels of free sugars, the low intake of omega-3 fats in the Western diet is contributing to the rise in type 2 diabetes in children and adults. According to the National Diet and Nutrition Survey every age group in the UK is exceeding the government's recommendations for free-sugar intake, with girls aged 11–18 and boys aged 4–10 consuming the most on average. This is the time not only when brains are undergoing rapid development but when future nutritional habits are being solidified.

How Can We Fix This?

Okay, so what do we know? We know that the brain depends on glucose, but that too much for too long can predispose us to high blood sugar and insulin insensitivity. So maintaining or restoring insulin sensitivity is key to avoiding the negative physical and mental consequences of hyperglycaemia. This can be achieved through dietary management, lifestyle factors like physical activity, or medications such as metformin which improve insulin sensitivity. One of the side effects of metformin use is B12 deficiency (see page 20), so patients taking this medication should have their blood levels checked regularly by their doctor.

One way of reducing the amount of sugar the country consumes would be for the government to order food manufacturers to reduce the quantity of sugar in their products. This system is called 'mandatory reformulation'. However, some, especially food manufacturers themselves, consider this to be a heavy-handed approach. Surely, having outlined all the serious health concerns, we can trust the food industry to 'do the right thing' and make voluntary changes to improve the nutritional profiles of their foods and protect the health of their customers?

No, friend, the food industry will fight for the right to promote foods high in fat, salt or sugar (HFSS) to children. Literally. See below.

KELLOGG'S

In 2019 the UK government undertook a public consultation on the inclusion of HFSS foods in supermarket volume promotions such as 'buy one get one free'. This was in response to the fact that overconsumption of HFSS foods contributes to weight gain, and volume sales promote increased purchase and thus increased consumption of these items.

The outcome was a programme of restrictions on the in-store promotion of HFSS foods, meaning that they cannot be placed in prominent positions such as the supermarket entrance or the highly profitable aisle ends. This included products like Kellogg's Frosties, Coco Pops and chocolate-filled Krave.

Rather than graciously accepting that the worsening health of the nation's children was a problem worth tackling, Kellogg's instead opted to take the government to court. No, really. Kellogg's took the Department of Health and Social Care to court. But here's the good part. The company were unable to deny that their products meet the criteria for HFSS foods. For example, Frosties (you know, the cereal with the cartoon tiger on the front) provide 87g of carbohydrates per 100g, of which 37g is

---

added sugar. In the UK a food is considered 'high sugar' if it contains more than 22.5g of sugar per 100g.

So instead they built their case around milk. To paraphrase: 'Most people have their cereal with milk,' they said, 'and if you include the nutritional properties of milk then our cereal is no longer junk food.'

The judge dismissed the claim.

The onus for reformulation must come from policy. Previously Kellogg's reformulated Coco Pops (the one with the cartoon monkey on the front) to contain 40 per cent less sugar so that it would no longer meet the criteria as a high-sugar food. Drinks manufacturers only reformulated their beverages to contain less sugar after the introduction of the sugar tax (see page 250). When dealing with multinational companies, profit (not consumer health) is king. The guaranteed way to effect change is to hit them in their pockets.

The bad news continues into adolescence. Just three weeks of low to moderate consumption of SSBs increased blood levels of the pro-inflammatory cytokine C-reactive protein by 60–109 per cent in healthy young men. We should be concerned about this effect on immune signalling because chronic inflammation is associated with a range of physical and mental health conditions such as heart disease, arthritis, depression and anxiety. High levels of circulating cytokines can impair the integrity of the blood-brain barrier (BBB), a highly selective layer of cells that prevents harmful substances crossing from the brain into the bloodstream (see page 201).

In a separate study, higher intake of SSBs was linked with lower brain volume and poorer cognitive performance. The researchers state that the effects on brain size of consuming 1–2 or more SSBs per day was equivalent to 1–2 years of brain aging. In terms of actual performance on cognitive tests it was likened to having a brain that was 6–11 years older. Excess sugar consumption can also alter neuronal activity in such a way as to increase the likelihood of experiencing depression, anxiety and panic.

Most adolescents know that sugary drinks have health risks. The likelihood of teens consuming them is largely driven by whether their parents do or not. A reminder that humans are rarely rational decision-makers, acting on the information provided. Our choices and behaviours are shaped by our environments.

A reminder that the NHS recommends:

- Children aged 4–6 should have no more than 19g of free sugars a day (five sugar cubes).
- Children aged 7–10 should have no more than 24g of free sugars a day (six sugar cubes).
- Adults should have no more than 30g of free sugars a day (roughly equivalent to seven sugar cubes).

A single can of a sugar-sweetened beverage can meet or exceed these limits. In the UK we are greatly overshooting the recommended safe sugar intake from SSBs. In fact, these beverages are a major contributor to the total free sugar for most adults. A 330ml can of original flavour Coca-Cola contains some 35g of sugar, which is over 100 per cent of the free sugar an adult should consume in a day.

So, through a range of mechanisms – reduced cellular energy availability, thiamine loss, vascular damage, worn-out and dysfunctional mitochondria and impaired omega-3 uptake – high blood glucose and diabetes set the scene for neurodegeneration, cognitive impairment and dementia on a national scale.

In May 2022 the then Secretary of State for Health and Social Care, Sajid Javid, announced an 'ambitious' ten-year strategy to tackle dementia, with a focus on prevention (which is our best hope of reducing rates of this condition). The well-known association between diabetes and dementia should have meant that one of his key targets was the improvement of children's diets. A truly ambitious plan would seek to: drastically improve the quality of school food; increase the affordability of fruits and vegetables, particularly for the poorest households; make the food environment more conducive to prompting brain-healthy choices by limiting children's exposure to HFSS food advertising. I would love to see cookery classes reintroduced for all children from years 7–10. Being able to feed yourself well and affordably is a life skill that we should be promoting in all children.

Unfortunately, on Tuesday, 5 July 2022, Mr Javid resigned from his post in protest at the conduct of the then prime minister, Boris Johnson. At the time of writing, it is not clear whether any of his successors will pick up the baton and follow through on his promise, but the early indications are not promising. As well as abandoning the health inequality white paper, the policy document published in September 2022 did not mention the word dementia (the leading cause of death in the UK) once. Nor was there any mention of 'food' or 'nutrition'.

A TALE OF TWO BRAINS

On Sundays Eleni would bring over a small tray of baklava (a syrup-drenched dessert). The family enjoyed one each after dinner. Otherwise, if she wanted something sweet after dinner her mother would give Anya a little cup of Greek yoghurt with a spoonful of honey stirred in, or a few grapes. Growing up she drank water with dinner as her mother had. Otherwise she drank milk or tea. Because she did not have them early in life or regularly, Anya did not develop a strong liking for sweet foods. The family's habit of only eating them after meals increases the likelihood that this is how Anya will consume these foods as an adult (rather than as between-meal snacks, for example). This habit of having sweet foods as part of or after a meal helped to keep Anya's blood sugar levels more constant. Not only did this support her mood (more on this later) but it reduced the risk of her developing hyperglycaemia. She also found it pretty easy to maintain a steady weight.

Conversely, Mia was weaned on sugar-sweetened foods and developed an early liking for them. She loved the rusk biscuits that she had been eating since she was six months old and continued to

eat them into toddlerhood (before transitioning to 'grown-up' biscuits). On days when she was very fussy Zoe would give her rusk
biscuits as it seemed to be the only thing that she would eat and at
least they had some goodness in them, she thought. Gradually, Mia
would eat more foods: baby yoghurts, bananas, mashed potato. Like
her mum she developed a reliance on ready meals. Zoe grew up
drinking her favourite orange squash. As a teenager, when she
started to become more conscious of her weight, she asked her mum
to switch to sugar-free squash. Around this time, she also adopted
the habit of skipping breakfast and just having an energy drink
instead. She knew she should drink more water but she found it very,
very boring. Having flavoured water helped a little bit but she would
often have a diet soda as she found them more refreshing.

Having developed an early liking for sweet foods Zoe is more
likely to consume them on a day-to-day basis. This risks chronically
elevating her blood glucose, which increases the chances of her later
developing diabetes, with the associated brain health risks.

CHAPTER 7

ULTRA-PROCESSED FOODS

WHAT DOES IT mean to be good? Most people would agree that it is not good to steal, to take something from someone else simply because you want it. But what about if you *need* it. Is a woman who steals a carton of baby formula from a supermarket to feed her child doing a bad thing? Is she a 'bad person'? I suspect that only the most fundamental moralists among us would condemn a mother for doing everything she could to feed her child. So we can see that our judgement of the 'goodness' or 'badness' of an action or behaviour is mediated by the contextual information. What is being stolen? By whom? For what purpose? Life is complicated and we must approach complicated subjects with the requisite nuance.

Now, food is complicated. I mean, really, really complicated. Not only does a single food item (such as an apple) contain hundreds, maybe thousands of compounds that vary by species, time/age of harvest, growing conditions, etc., but each of these compounds can interact with our bodies, our genes and our microbiomes in incalculable ways. And our bodies will each require different things at different times. Breast milk is the ideal complete food for a newborn baby but it's not going to get a 26-year-old very far. Our nutritional needs vary with age, sex, activity levels, health status, genetics, time of year, geographic location, etc. For that reason we should consider the discipline of nutritional research every bit as complex as the study of genetics. Maybe even more so because nutrients can interact with genes! Therefore, anyone who tells you that there is one ideal way to eat for everyone simply does not know what they are talking about.

This issue of 'good' and 'bad' food invariably comes up when discussing nutrition and mental health. You may have noticed that I haven't called any food 'bad' in this book. That's because, like our formula-stealing mother, the 'goodness' or 'badness' of a food is relative to the context. If I have a healthy diet (for example, I eat a lot of fruits and vegetables, wholegrains, nuts, seeds, etc.) then one piece of chocolate is not going to strain my system or do me harm; if 80 per cent of my diet is chocolate, I'm likely to be malnourished. So the problem isn't the chocolate per se, it's the proportion and where it sits in my overall diet.

Broadly, this is the perspective that I want to take with this chapter because we are about to dip our toes into some of the most complicated and contentious features of the modern food environment: ultra-processed foods (UPFs). In fact, even settling on a definition is a slightly controversial position. Many people have tried to offer simple heuristics for how to spot and avoid UPFs:

- Don't eat anything your grandmother wouldn't have recognised as food.
- Don't buy anything with more than five ingredients.
- Don't eat it if sugar is one of the top three ingredients.
- If you can't pronounce it, don't eat it.

You can see what all of these are getting at. Some combination of 'eat wholefoods', 'limit sugar' and 'avoid industrial additives'. All reasonable positions but all have limits to their utility. Depending on your background, your grandmother might not have recognised sashimi, ackee or kajmak, which all happen to be nutritious wholefoods. So maybe making your grandmother the arbiter of your food choices isn't the ideal approach. Sorry, Nana.

If any of you have completed distance runs – 10k, half-marathon, marathon, that kind of thing – either along the route, and certainly in the goody bag, you will have encountered some kind of glucose-sweetened bar or gel. Now, for a weekday breakfast en route to your desk job, perhaps this is not the most nutritious choice, but if you have just completed intense exercise then, frankly, this is probably exactly what you need.

Many people would struggle pronouncing docosahexaenoic acid, but I just expended a few thousand words explaining why it's so important for brain health. So, simple one-liners are inadequate tools for identifying UPFs. We need something more comprehensive.

Recently, a research group attempted to codify principles of what constitutes a UPF. Called the NOVA classification, they divide foods into one of four groups based on the nature, extent and purpose of food processing.

The NOVA Classification

1.	Unprocessed or minimally processed foods	Unprocessed (or natural) foods are edible parts of plants (seeds, fruits, leaves, stems, roots) or of animals (muscle, offal, eggs, milk), and also fungi, algae and water.
		Minimally processed foods are natural foods altered by processes such as the removal of inedible or unwanted parts, drying, crushing, grinding, fractioning, filtering, roasting, boiling, pasteurisation, refrigeration, freezing, placing in containers, vacuum-packaging or non-alcoholic fermentation. None of these processes adds substances such as salt, sugar, oils or fats. The main purpose of the processes used in the production of group 1 foods is to extend the life of unprocessed foods, allowing their storage for longer use, such as chilling, freezing, drying and pasteurising.
		Other purposes include facilitating or diversifying food preparation, such as in the removal of inedible parts and fractioning of vegetables, the crushing or grinding of seeds, the roasting of coffee beans or tea leaves and the fermentation of milk to make yoghurt.
		Group 1 foods include fresh, squeezed, chilled, frozen or dried fruits and leafy and root vegetables; grains; legumes; starchy roots and tubers such as potatoes and cassava; meat, poultry, fish and seafood, whole or in the form of steaks, fillets and other cuts, or chilled or frozen; eggs; milk, pasteurised or powdered; fresh or pasteurised fruit or vegetable juices without added sugar, sweeteners or flavours; spices and herbs; dried mixed fruits, granola made from cereals, nuts and dried fruits with no added sugar, honey or oil.

2.	Processed culinary ingredients	These are substances obtained directly from group 1 foods or from nature by processes such as pressing, refining, grinding, milling and spray-drying. The purpose of processing here is to make products used in home and restaurant kitchens to prepare, season and cook group 1 foods and to make with them varied and enjoyable homemade dishes, soups and broths, breads, preserves, salads, drinks, desserts and other culinary preparations.
		Group 2 items are rarely consumed in the absence of group 1 foods. Examples are salt mined or from seawater; sugar and molasses obtained from cane or beet; honey extracted from combs and syrup from maple trees; vegetable oils crushed from olives or seeds; butter and lard obtained from milk and pork; and starches extracted from corn and other plants.
3.	Processed foods	These are relatively simple products made by adding sugar, oil, salt or other group 2 substances to group 1 foods. Most processed foods have two or three ingredients. Processes include various preservation or cooking methods, and, in the case of breads and cheese, non-alcoholic fermentation. The main purpose of the manufacture of processed foods is to increase the durability of group 1 foods, or to modify or enhance their sensory qualities.
		Typical examples of processed foods are canned or bottled vegetables, fruits and legumes; salted or sugared nuts and seeds; salted, cured or smoked meats; canned fish; fruits in syrup; cheeses and unpackaged freshly made breads. Processed foods may contain additives used to preserve their original properties or to resist microbial contamination. Examples are fruits in syrup with added antioxidants and dried, salted meats with added preservatives.
4.	Ultra-processed food and drink products	This groups gets its name from the fact that the constituent parts have gone through several methods of industrial processing to achieve the end product. The research group describe these foods as 'energy-dense, high in unhealthy types of fat, refined starches, free sugars and salt and poor sources of protein, dietary fibre and micronutrients. Ultra-processed products are made to be hyper-palatable and attractive, with long shelf life, and able to be consumed anywhere, any time. Their formulation, presentation and marketing often promote overconsumption', and they add that 'the ever-increasing production and consumption of these products is a *world crisis*'.
		Ultra-processed food and drink products are industrial formulations typically with five or more, and usually many, ingredients. Such ingredients often include those also used in processed foods, such as sugar, oils, fats, salt, antioxidants, stabilisers and preservatives. Ingredients only found in ultra-processed products include substances not commonly used in culinary preparations, and additives whose purpose is to imitate the sensory qualities of

group 1 foods or to disguise undesirable sensory qualities of the final product. Group 1 foods are a small proportion of or are even absent from ultra-processed products. Substances only found in ultra-processed products include some directly extracted from foods, such as casein, lactose, whey and gluten, and some derived from further processing of food constituents, such as hydrogenated or interesterified oils, hydrolysed proteins, soy protein isolate, maltodextrin, invert sugar and high-fructose corn syrup. Classes of additive only found in ultra-processed products include dyes and other colours, colour stabilisers, flavours, flavour enhancers, non-sugar sweeteners and processing aids such as carbonating, firming, bulking and anti-bulking, de-foaming, anti-caking and glazing agents, emulsifiers, sequestrants and humectants.

Several industrial processes with no domestic equivalents are used in the manufacture of ultra-processed products, such as extrusion and moulding, and pre-processing for frying. The main purpose of industrial ultra-processing is to create products that are ready to eat, to drink or to heat, liable to replace both unprocessed or minimally processed foods that are naturally ready to consume, such as fruits and nuts, milk and water, and freshly prepared drinks, dishes, desserts and meals.

Examples of typical ultra-processed products are: carbonated drinks; sweet or savoury packaged snacks; ice cream, chocolate, candies (confectionery); mass-produced packaged breads and buns; margarines and spreads; cookies (biscuits), pastries, cakes and cake mixes; breakfast 'cereals', 'cereal' and 'energy' bars; 'energy' drinks; milk drinks, 'fruit' yoghurts and 'fruit' drinks; cocoa drinks; meat and chicken extracts and 'instant' sauces; infant formulas, follow-on milks, other baby products; 'health' and 'slimming' products such as powdered or 'fortified' meal and dish substitutes; and many ready-to-heat products including pre-prepared pies and pasta and pizza dishes; poultry and fish 'nuggets' and 'sticks', sausages, burgers, hot dogs, and other reconstituted meat products, and powdered and packaged 'instant' soups, noodles and desserts.

This classification was proposed because, in the last 50 years, food has become much more complex. Whereas in the 1950s and 1960s (when dietary guidelines were just being developed) you might have had the option of consuming an orange or a glass of freshly squeezed orange juice, now you can have freshly squeezed orange juice or juice from concentrate with or without the pulp, orange juice drink, orange soda with or without sugar, orange-flavoured energy drinks, orange-flavoured vitamin water, orange-flavoured protein water (a real thing), orange-flavoured water with added magnesium, orange squash sweetened with sugar or orange squash with the following ingredients:

> *Water, Orange Fruit from Concentrate (10%), Acid (Citric Acid), Acidity Regulator (Sodium Citrate), Natural Orange Flavouring with other Natural Flavourings, Preservatives (Potassium Sorbate, Sodium Metabisulphite), Sweeteners (Acesulfame K, Sucralose), Stabilisers (Cellulose Gum, Sucrose Acetate Isobutyrate), Emulsifier (Glycerol Esters of Wood Rosins), Natural Colour (Carotenes).*

Now, all of these ingredients are generally recognised as safe (or GRAS – a legal definition) in terms of human metabolism, but what is clear is that the nutrition that you attain from consuming an orange is far superior to what you can achieve from a glass of this squash made up as per the manufacturer's instructions:

One medium orange	Robinsons Orange Squash No Added Sugar
58kcal/243kJ	3kcal/13kJ
1.3g protein	0.08g salt
0.3g fat	Contains negligible amounts of fat,
13.1g carbohydrate	saturates, carbohydrate, sugars and protein
1.9g fibre	
195mg potassium	
53mcg folate	
83mg vitamin C	

If you want hydration and the delicious taste of oranges, nutritionally you would be better off eating an orange and drinking a glass of water, or even adding a little fresh orange juice to your water bottle.

The UK leads the way in the consumption of UPFs across Europe. In the UK currently 55 per cent of adults' calories are from ultra-processed foods, mostly from baked goods (cakes and biscuits), confectionery, processed meats and soft drinks, and that figure is growing. Americans are slightly ahead of us, with ultra-processed food and drinks (UPFDs) making up 57 per cent of their daily calories. At last count Italians consumed the fewest UPFDs, with these items making up just 14 per cent of their daily calories. Though risk is not wholly attributable to diet, it is interesting to note that dementia is the eighth leading cause of death in Italy, despite the Italians having a longer life expectancy than the British.

Though one glass of squash isn't going to kill you, there are reasonable grounds to be concerned about the majority of our diets consisting of these industrialised foods:

1. The nature of processing means that brain-healthy nutrients – vitamins, minerals, essential fats and fibre – are lost (see page 94 for the example of thiamine).
2. Fewer antioxidants. Recall that brain fats are prone to oxidation, which increases inflammation. Nutrients found in fresh fruit and vegetables, such as vitamin C, beta-carotene and lycopene, can mitigate ROS.
3. In order to extend shelf life and palatability, additional sugar and fats are added, which may have negative consequences for brain health.
4. Finally, and most importantly, the convenience of these foods means that they increasingly displace more nutritious but more labour-intensive foods from our diets. For example, during the same period that US consumption of UPFDs increased from 53.5 to 57 per cent of daily energy intake, consumption of minimally processed foods dropped from 32.7 to 27.4 per cent.

It is this nutritional displacement, I think, that explains why high UPF consumption is linked to worsening brain health, and actively fuelling our mental health crisis.

The more our diets are made up of UPFDs, the lower our daily nutrient intake. A 2015 Brazilian study that assessed the diets of over 32,898 individuals over the age of ten showed that the consumption of UPFs was inversely correlated to the intake of vitamins B12, D, E, niacin (B3), pyridoxine (B6), copper, iron, phosphorus, magnesium, selenium and zinc. A more recent Mexican study of 10,000 people aged over one year found the same thing: the higher the consumption of UPFs, the lower the intake of B vitamins, vitamins C and E, and minerals. Omega-3s, vitamins A, B12, C and E, calcium and zinc were lower in a cohort of Colombian children, though folate and iron were higher as many ultra-processed foods are fortified with these nutrients.

This is particularly bad news for our hard-working brains which require a constant supply of nutrients to function properly. And this is beginning to be borne out in the research. A French prospective cohort study of over 26,000 people, who were assessed at baseline and then followed up around five years later, found a significant association between UPF consumption and depression risk. A study of 14,000 Spanish university graduates found the same thing: those individuals in the highest quintile of UPF consumption had the greatest risk of developing depression in the intervening decade.

As UPFs begin to displace more nutrient-dense wholefoods we are starting to see evidence of negative effects on brain and mental health. A 2021 study published in *BMJ Nutrition, Prevention & Health* of over 8,000 UK children found an association between higher consumption of fruits and vegetables and self-reported mental wellbeing. For secondary-school children they saw a linear or dose-response pattern; that is, for each extra portion of fruit and veg consumed (measured up to 'five or more') their mental wellbeing score went up. Sure, but that probably means they came from wealthier, less stressed households too, right? Yes, that is probably true, but when the researchers adjusted the analysis to account for factors such as alcohol consumption, smoking status, income markers such as whether they had their own bed and adverse events such as bullying or not feeling safe at home, the association held – more fruit and veg was linked to better mental health. But if you need more convincing, we can look at the brains of people on Western vs wholefood/minimally processed diets.

In a longitudinal study that looked at the brains of older people over the course of four years there was a direct relationship between diet quality and hippocampal size; the healthier the diet, the larger the area of the brain's memory centre, which is a good thing as it generally means there are more connections (cognitive reserve). A separate study showed negative effects on the brain emerge *within days* on a Western

UPF diet. In this study 110 healthy people, who typically ate a nutritious diet, were asked to eat a Western-type diet for just a week. Within that week they were asked to eat two Belgian waffles for breakfast on four of the days and consume a takeaway meal twice. Compared to a control group, the Western-style diet group suffered impairments in hippocampal-dependent learning and memory and poorer appetite control. The declines in learning and memory correlated to the degree of impaired appetite control, indicating that damage to the hippocampus underlined these changes. So it is a vicious cycle: the more these foods are consumed, the more damage to the hippocampus, the worse the appetite controls, the more these foods are consumed . . .

I don't know about you but I find that terrifying. The hippocampus is the part of the brain that is substantially damaged in Alzheimer's disease. The fact that measurable brain damage can be induced by just a few days on a diet that many people eat habitually should be a cause for considerable concern.

And the picture for the rapidly developing brains of children is, frankly, alarming. A recent 19-year prospective study of the diets of over 9,000 UK children and young people aged 7–24 found that one in five were consuming over 78 per cent of their daily calories from UPFs. The main categories of UPFDs in the high consumption group were fruit-based or fizzy drinks, ready meals and ready-made cakes and biscuits. The authors also found a dose-response relationship between UPFDs and adiposity (fat accumulation) over time – that is, the higher the proportion of UPFDs in the diet, the greater the proportion of body fat. This study also showed that the dietary patterns that were established in childhood persisted into adulthood. Commenting on the results, Professor Christopher Millett, NIHR Professor of Public Health at Imperial College London, said:

Through a lack of regulation, and enabling the low cost and ready availability of these foods, we are damaging our children's long-term health. We urgently need effective policy change to redress the balance, to protect the health of children and reduce the proportion of these foods in their diet.

And, as Professor Millett mentions, cost is a major consideration in the promotion and adoption of healthier diets. Nutritious, fresh foods are, calorie-for-calorie, at least three times more expensive than their ultra-processed, industrially produced counterparts. Research by the Food Foundation, a charity that campaigns for changes to food policy to make healthy diets more accessible, showed that in order to meet the recommendations of the government's 'Eatwell' guidelines, the poorest fifth of UK households would need to spend 47 per cent of their disposable income compared to just 11 per cent for the wealthiest households. As fuel and energy costs rise, wealthier households have a sufficient cushion of disposable income to absorb the increase. For the poorest, there is simply less money left over for food. And with food prices one of the main contributing factors to our record inflation rates, the diets of the poorest families are put under unbearable pressure.

And the evidence is that the first casualties of this pressure are fruit and vegetables. The consumption of fruit and vegetables is directly linked to their affordability. Children from poorer households are less likely to consume fresh produce than their wealthier classmates. A 2014 government survey found that three times as many boys (aged 5–15) from the most deprived backgrounds ate absolutely no fruit and veg compared to the least deprived boys.

In response to similar nutritional inequalities in the US, the Department of Agriculture introduced the Fresh Fruit and Vegetable Program (FFVP), which, as the name suggests, provides fresh fruit and veg to schools in areas of deprivation – that is, the schools with the highest proportion of children in receipt of free or reduced-cost meals. The stated goals of the FFVP are 'to introduce children to fresh fruits and vegetables, to include new and different varieties, and to increase overall acceptance and consumption of fresh, unprocessed produce among children. The FFVP also encourages healthier school environments by promoting nutrition education.' As part of the programme fresh fruit and vegetables are offered outside of the main mealtimes (i.e. as snacks). The project is federally funded, with schools receiving between $50 and $75 per child per school year, which the schools can use to purchase produce from wholesalers, supermarkets or smaller local providers and growers. An impact assessment found that children who participated in the programme consumed more beta-carotene, vitamins A and C and fibre, compared to non-participants. When asked, 97 per cent of the students said they wanted the FFVP to continue at their school.

The UK's School Fruit and Vegetable Scheme (SFVS) entitles all children aged 4–6 attending state-funded schools to one piece of fruit or veg per day. However, the scheme has been criticised for the lack of quality of the produce – hard, underripe pears and carrots sweating in bags for days – actually putting children off eating it. In his independent review of the National Food Strategy, published in July 2021, Henry Dimbleby recommended doubling government funding of the scheme from £40 million to £80 million, and delivering the money directly to schools so that they could purchase higher-quality produce for themselves. He also recommended extending the provision to infant schools. However, there is no evidence that these recommendations are being actioned. Conversely, the scheme appears to be constantly 'under review', raising concerns about its longevity.

TAKE ACTION

Ask your MP to commit to the long-term security of the School Fruit and Vegetable Scheme.

Go to https://www.theyworkforyou.com/mps/ to find the name and contact details of your local MP. Be polite.

What about Functional Foods?

Always resourceful, the food industry is now offering us solutions for problems that, arguably, they have created, in the form of functional foods. Functional foods are a subtype of UPFs that have had particular nutrients added back in. For example, a butter-like spread with added plant-derived chemicals to help reduce cholesterol, or tea bags with added vitamins. The market, which was valued at $180,843.73

million in 2021, is booming and growth is expected to continue well into 2027. It's kind of brilliant. They produce, heavily market and sell foods that are nutrient-poor and then sell you the nutrients back in *another product*. It is business genius. In the context of a nutrient-poor diet high in UPFs, functional foods have some benefit, particularly for fussy or picky eaters who might only consume a limited range of foods. However, there are hundreds, probably thousands of nutrients in wholefoods that have not been isolated by food scientists so simply cannot be added to manufactured foods.

Boris and the BOGOFs

The pandemic occasioned many of us to reconsider and revalue our health. Initially belligerent about the potential risk of the virus, the then British prime minister, Boris Johnson, is reported to have missed five emergency COBRA meetings where responses to the impending pandemic were being discussed and planned. His lack of awareness and regard for even the most basic disease-control measures was made clear when, on 3 March 2020, he told a room full of reporters, 'I'm shaking hands continuously. I was at a hospital the other night where . . . there were a few coronavirus patients and I shook hands with everybody, you'll be pleased to know. And I continue to shake hands.' Twenty days later the UK was placed under its first lockdown in which the public were told we had to stay at home except to shop for basic necessities, exercise, or to attend medical appointments. Gatherings of more than two people in public were forbidden.

The early days of lockdown felt otherworldly. Seemingly overnight so much that we had considered to be safe and true was turned on its head. Offices were closed, children sent home from school. There were queues outside the supermarket and shortages on their shelves. And, as we watched news stories of hard-hit countries, the true scale of the pandemic began to dawn. Hospitals struggled to cope with wave after wave of patients requiring ventilation and intensive care. Nurses called in to radio programmes and spoke tearfully of feeling burned-out and helpless.

UNDERLYING HEALTH CONDITIONS

It was around this time that an unlikely phrase – 'underlying health condition' – soared in online search popularity. Early cross-sectional research was indicating that certain health conditions increased the risk of being hospitalised with coronavirus. Consequently, the government released a list of those at greater risk from Covid-19:

- Anyone aged 70 or older (regardless of medical conditions)
- Anyone under 70 with an underlying health condition listed below (i.e. anyone instructed to get a flu jab as an adult each year on medical grounds):
  - chronic (long-term) respiratory diseases, such as asthma, chronic obstructive pulmonary disease (COPD), emphysema or bronchitis
  - chronic heart disease, such as heart failure
  - chronic kidney disease
  - chronic liver disease, such as hepatitis
  - chronic neurological conditions, such as Parkinson's disease, motor neurone disease, multiple sclerosis (MS), a learning disability or cerebral palsy
  - diabetes
  - problems with your spleen – for example, sickle cell disease or if you have had your spleen removed
  - a weakened immune system as the result of conditions such as HIV and AIDS, or medicines such as steroid tablets or chemotherapy
  - being seriously overweight (a BMI of 40 or above)
- Those who are pregnant

The helplessness was, I think, a major part of the shared experience of the pandemic. People responded to this powerlessness in different ways. Some obsessively tracked the numbers: positive tests, hospitalisations, the death count. Some munificently challenged their own helplessness by helping others. Still others tried to stave off feelings of vulnerability by reducing or eliminating their risk factors. A million people found the motivation to quit smoking after we learned that smokers had a higher chance of both contracting the virus and an increased risk of developing severe symptoms when they did. I clearly remember patients of mine who were carrying extra weight feeling very frightened that they were 'putting themselves at risk' when higher body fat was linked to increased Covid-19 mortality.

During this time sales of dietary supplements skyrocketed as anxious individuals sought nutritional support for immunity and general health. In March 2020, as many countries began to introduce partial and full national lockdowns to slow the spread of the virus, sales of multivitamins rose by 51 per cent in America, by 63 per cent in the UK and around 50 per cent in France.

On 27 March 2020, the prime minister declared that he had tested positive for Covid-19 and entered a period of self-isolation. By Sunday, 5 April, he still had symptoms and was admitted to London's St Thomas' Hospital, just a stone's throw from his Downing Street residence, as a 'precautionary measure'. By the next day he had been transferred to the intensive care unit, where he remained for three nights. On Saturday, 11 April, Mr Johnson announced that he owed his life to the care of the hospital staff.

In Charles Dickens's *A Christmas Carol*, it is the visit from the third and final ghost that cements the transformation of miserly Ebenezer Scrooge's attitude to the world. On seeing his name on the neglected gravestone and the absence of affection from those attending his funeral, Scrooge promises that he is a changed man who will keep the spirit of Christmas, of generosity and kindness to others, in his heart all year round. On his release from hospital the prime minister seemed to have had a similar revelation. Describing himself as 'too fat' when he was admitted to hospital, Boris Johnson was inspired not only to transform his own health but to introduce important new measures aimed at reducing the growing rates of overweight and obesity in UK children and adults.

And he quickly got to work drafting his plan of action. In a press release published on 27 July 2020 the government announced a new 'obesity strategy', which included key nutrition-related targets:

- A ban on TV and online adverts for food high in fat, sugar and salt before 9pm.
- Legislation to end deals like BOGOFs – 'buy one get one free' – on foods high in salt, sugar and fat.
- Calories to be displayed on restaurant menus to help people make lower-calorie choices when eating out.
- A new campaign to help people lose weight, get active and eat better after the Covid-19 'wake-up call'.

In addition there was to be a consultation on whether to list the hidden 'liquid calories' on alcohol.

The full strategy document (my emphasis) outlined the rationale behind these decisions:

> Many people have tried to lose weight but struggle in the face of endless prompts to eat – on TV and on the high street. In supermarkets, special offers and promotions tempt us to buy foods that are not on the shopping list but are hard to resist. When we eat out, we have little information about how many calories are in the food we are offered. *We are biologically programmed to eat and when we are bombarded by advertisements and promotions for food* – it's hard to eat healthily, especially if we are busy or tired or stressed . . .
>
> A survey from 2018 shows that around 43% of all food and drink products located in prominent areas, such as store entrances, checkouts, and aisle ends were for sugary foods and drinks and less than 1% of food and drink products promoted in high-profile locations in store were fruit or vegetables. *The location of products within stores can also significantly affect our purchases.* For example, end-of-aisle displays have been shown to increase soft drink sales by just over 50%.

Promotions like buy one get one free (BOGOF) which encourage us to buy more to get the deal appear to be mechanisms to help shoppers save money, however data shows that they *actually increase the amount we spend by almost 20% by encouraging people to buy more than they need or intended to buy in the first place. These are not 'good deals' for our wallet or our health* . . .

Current advertising restrictions for HFSS products during children's TV and other programming of particular appeal to children are *insufficient to protect children* from seeing a significant amount of unhealthy food adverts on TV, and don't account for the increasing amount of time they are spending online. *Research shows that exposing children to these adverts can increase the amount of food children eat and shape their preferences from a young age.*

This very clear statement, from the government's own research, emphasises how powerful the influence of advertising and the food environment is on our food choices and our health.

However, unlike Scrooge, who we are given to believe kept his promise, Johnson's Damascene conversion was startlingly short-lived. In May 2022 the UK government abandoned its plans to ban supermarket 'buy one get one free' deals on high fat, sugar and salt foods. Johnson claimed that the decision to 'delay' implementation was driven by a desire to soften the blow of the 'cost of living squeeze', the predictably euphemistic term for the brutal combination of record inflation, stagnant wages, and soaring energy prices which really means that more households will be pushed into poverty and food insecurity. This specious justification fails to explain why he also ditched the proposal to implement a 9pm watershed on the advertisement of ultra-processed and fast foods, a move that could only result in reduced sales and more money saved. No, this flimsy justification simply doesn't hold water.

First, as noted in the government's own fiscal analysis of the impact of volume-based deals, they do not save shoppers money: they make us buy more. The justification provided directly contradicted the word and spirit of his own policy.

What's going on? In a candid article for *The Times* newspaper published on 16 May 2022, former Conservative Party leader Lord William Hague explained: 'Under pressure from some Conservative MPs, some of whom have been threatening to write letters of no confidence in Boris Johnson unless they get their way, ministers have retreated from banning buy-one-get-one-free deals and from imposing a watershed of 9pm on junk food advertising.' During this period Boris Johnson and other members of his Cabinet and household were under scrutiny for ignoring lockdown rules and throwing parties in Downing Street while thousands of people around the country were forced to say final goodbyes to loved ones over video call due to the government-imposed limits on public gatherings. The devastating hypocrisy was understandably unpopular, putting Johnson's position at risk and opening up the possibility of a leadership challenge.

The rather unpalatable conclusion is that the prime minister was more concerned with securing his temporary position at the top of the heap than investing in the health of future generations. Moreover, everyone around him knew it and used his desperation to remain in post to control him. Meanwhile, other countries have taken decisive action. Brazil's national nutrition guidelines now explicitly caution against the consumption of UPFs and even warn people to be wary of food advertising:

> *The purpose of advertising is to increase product sales, and not to inform or educate people. Be critical and teach children to be critical of all forms of food advertising and marketing.*

UK public health campaigners were understandably disappointed and angry. I spoke to Jenny Rosborough, who is the former campaign manager for Action on Sugar and the current Head of Nutrition at Jamie Oliver Limited, in her role as a Consultant Public Health Nutritionist:

JR: *The narrative that the government have given is to do with 'cost of living' and industry not being ready. Obviously, the marketing restrictions have nothing to do with the cost of living and, actually, price promotion doesn't either, which is what is really frustrating. They're pushing this narrative about keeping these BOGOFs because of 'cost of living', they want to 'support families' when all the evidence, even their own impact assessments, shows that it just encourages people to spend more and actually businesses can just reduce the prices and make each individual thing cheaper. That was never taken away. It was just those buy-one-get-one-frees that make you buy more and eat more and spend more. The actual reason was that Boris was being threatened with 'votes of no confidence' because of all of the ongoing scandals and he had to keep people on side to keep his position. So obviously . . . we know that they prioritise their own egos over public health.*

This is the other thing: [how] to make it matter to people that are not suffering the consequences of the decisions they have to make. When they need to prioritise, 'What do I do? Do I help put food on the table for that family, or do I make sure that I'm still popular in the playground?' It's very easy for them to prioritise being popular in the playground.

KW: *What are your concerns about the health of UK children or adults?*

JR: *I think it's just generally seeing the impact of the Westernised ultra-processed, typically energy-dense, nutrient-poor foods. And I don't want to just talk about obesity because when you do that, it looks like these policies [aren't] relevant for the whole population. And they are because, ultimately, it's about a lack of nutrient density. So obesity might be one thing, but lack of nutrients . . . well, lack of food in general for some people but especially nutritious food.*

But the overriding thing there is that we are seeing the impact of the foods that we're eating on various health outcomes and it doesn't seem to be a matter of urgency for government. And yet it is something that could be preventable in the right environment. And I think that's frustrating for a country as advanced as the UK, because we are one of the worst when it comes to consumption of ultra-processed foods and how we let it get to that is really depressing.

KW: How did we let it get to that?

JR: That is a good question. I think it's a lot to do with food culture. Going back to the adverts and the marketing and advertisers proposing 'solutions' for us. We are sold a certain way of eating and we need a whole cultural shift, I think, and that can only really happen with legislation. I think that's the main thing, and then there is obviously the food insecurity. We know that more socially deprived families are disproportionately impacted. And so this is where it becomes way out of the Department of Health's control. This is where it has to be a systemic government approach that takes all of that into account.

One of the key things is about there being a lot of short-sightedness with PMs. They just want to be popular in their short cycle and then someone else is there. And that's really difficult because you need things in place now that are going to help in 20 years' time, but they're not going to get the credit for that.

Health professionals, campaigners, preconception and infant health researchers, that is, the people on the ground, at the front line, seeing patients every day, are united in saying that in order to improve child health (i.e. the health of the future of the nation) changes must be made to the ways in which food is marketed and priced. For one brief, shining moment Boris Johnson agreed with this too. But then he went back to thinking about himself. What we see is the abandoning of a public health policy for completely self-serving reasons. But it gets worse. Not only does the delay of this strategy due to the 'cost of living squeeze' not make fiscal sense, it's also worse for the health of the nation in several ways because the secondary outcome of buying more is that people eat more. So this 'delay' in the implementation of the strategy will not save people money and will contribute to worse physical and mental health outcomes for the most vulnerable in our society. These harms are multiplied by the physical and mental effects of poverty itself.

Already in May 2022 parents and older people were reporting cutting back on food or skipping meals to save money. This, of course, carries the risk of malnutrition. Less disposable income could also mean that people go out less, perhaps to save money on fuel or other transport costs. While the pandemic showed us that phone and video calls are a valuable resource, older people might struggle to use these technologies. Poorer nutrition and reduced social interaction are known risk factors for neurodegeneration. But there are also risks for younger people, and they have to do with the interaction between stress, eating and fat storage, as seen in the chapter on sugar (see page 87).

In experimental studies, when people are primed to feel anxious about their social position, they consume more calories. In this fascinating British study the experimenters artificially induced feelings of inequality and poverty. They did this by having the participants read one of two paragraphs that either described people in their society as being able to cover their living costs (the wealthy condition) or living from hand to mouth (poverty condition). They were then asked to write a few lines about how similar they were to the people they had just read about. Later, they were served some snacks under the pretence of a taste test. In the analysis they found that people induced to feel poor ate 54 per cent more calories that the wealthy group. Additionally, people who self-reported being of a lower socioeconomic group and feeling anxious about being looked down on also ate significantly more. Why would this happen? Because feelings of poverty trigger a scarcity response. To your brain scarcity means 'famine' and your anti-famine strategy kicks into motion. Eat more, store energy, get through the hard times.

Note that this is not a conscious choice. These participants had no idea that thinking about their social standing was causing them to eat more. Rather, it was an *automatic, unconscious and, for that reason, uncontrollable* response to the stress of, in this case, imagined poverty. Information that indicates scarcity is coming elicits this response. So we should expect that the 'cost of living crisis' will be accompanied by increased consumption and the associated health risks.

Remember, too, that we also find sweet, salty, highly palatable foods tastier and more pleasurable when we are stressed. This 'increased tastiness' might be part of the same mechanism: your brain makes these energy-dense foods taste better so that you are inclined to eat more of them to build up your fat stores. But it could also relate to the limited opportunities for pleasure that people are faced with when they have less money. You might not be able to take a day off work, go on holiday or buy some new clothes, but you can stretch to a chocolate bar that will provide a few moments of pleasure, a temporary relief from the stress of deprivation and hardship.

Conclusion

Though controversy remains over their exact definition, the growing scientific consensus is that our high consumption of UPFs is causing us harm. Not only do they displace more nutrient-dense foods in the diet but they are linked to harmful brain changes and impaired appetite control. However, these highly palatable foods are extremely profitable to food manufacturers. They have no incentive to make them healthier. Truly 'bold leadership' would mean a government that prioritises long-term public health over personal advancement.

Successive Conservative governments have failed to implement food policies that would meaningfully improve the food environment for the most vulnerable. Most recently Boris Johnson chose to sacrifice public health for personal political gain. The importance of having a policy is that most people do not know that what they are eating is UPF. Not only is the nature of food manufacture rather complex but legislation that allows food manufacturers to label their products as high in one or other nutrients means that many people will simply not realise how lacking in nutrients their diet is. This is of particular concern when it comes to children, teens and adolescents, whose brains are still developing but who are some of the highest consumers of ultra-processed foods.

A TALE OF TWO BRAINS

Anya's breakfast would vary. Sometimes she would have cornflakes with a sliced banana on top. On other days, toast and a boiled egg or slices of cheese, some fresh tomato and a few olives. In the winter she would have porridge because her *yiayia* Eleni had always told her it would help to keep her warm. Anya qualified for free school meals (FSM). Various things were on offer – hot dogs on Monday, burgers on Wednesday, but she usually chose something that was similar to what she grew up eating, like meatballs in sauce with rice or fish fillet with potato wedges and vegetables, or a jacket potato and a fruit pot.

Anya didn't have much trouble concentrating at school (unless the lesson was really boring) and made steady progress academically. She was placed in the top set for maths and was predicted good grades for her exams.

Most mornings Mia would have a bowl of cornflakes, rice pops or wheat biscuits for breakfast, with milk and sugar. Her mum would prepare lunch for her, which usually consisted of a cheese or ham sandwich on white bread, a packet of crisps and a two-finger KitKat alongside a carton of juice or squash. When she was older, if she ate school lunches, she would usually opt for a slice of pizza and shared her chips with a friend. At home she ate spaghetti bolognese, beans on toast, chicken nuggets, frozen burgers and oven chips or potato wedges.

Mia often had difficulty focusing in class, especially in the mornings. She would find herself distracted or just a bit irritable. Her teachers found this frustrating because they felt she was able but complained that she didn't 'apply herself'. Mia found this hurtful as she wasn't doing it intentionally. She didn't do badly at school but she never really felt that she reached her full potential and this made her doubt her abilities when applying for jobs. She also had bouts of low mood that started around the age of 16 and persisted throughout her twenties.

Anya's habitual diet was predominantly low-processed (groups 1–3 on the NOVA classification). In contrast, much of Mia's diet would be considered ultra-processed (indeed, the baby biscuits she was weaned on are an ultra-processed product). Her intake of free sugars was higher and her consumption of fibre, fresh fruits and vegetables (and consequently vitamins and minerals) was lower than Anya's. Evidence indicates that greater adherence to a minimally processed diet during childhood and adolescence is associated with greater self-reported wellbeing, enhanced mood and less psychological distress, which would account for Anya's steady mood and Mia's greater tendency to irritability and poor concentration. We will discuss the link between nutrition and children's behaviour in the chapter on nutrition and the cycle of poverty.

Finally, for children in receipt of free school meals, school lunch is an important source of nutrients. For many children it is the only hot meal they will have all day, which means we should ensure that these meals are nutritious and satisfying.

CHAPTER 8

PSYCHOBIOTICS

I STARTED TO make my own fermented foods over a decade ago.
I was partly inspired by my long-extent spirit of self-sufficiency. At 12
years old, when I realised that baked beans were just beans, tomatoes
and spices I decided I could make them just as well myself. I have a
vague recollection of slightly hard (impatient) beans in an otherwise
successful effort. My other incentive was the growing body of research
evidence indicating that this thing called the microbiome could have a
material effect on not just the brain's functions but its structure. Since
then the scientific and commercial interest in the microscopic inhabit-
ants of our colons has exploded. While the researchers caution that we
know perhaps just 1 per cent of what there is to learn about what the
microbiome is, how it functions, how it communicates with the brain
and what a 'healthy' microbiome actually looks like, commercial enti-
ties are already offering apps claiming to provide personalised advice
on what to eat and what to avoid to optimise your health. So what is
the microbiome and what can we say about its role in – specifically for
our purposes – brain structure and mental health?

Technically, I should specify that I am talking about the gut microbiome since we are discovering that almost all our bodily nooks,
crannies and crevices are populated by their own microbial communities. The vaginal microbiome, for example, helps to maintain a healthy,
slightly acidic pH, which is why practices such as douching can lead to

the development of bacterial vaginosis, an overgrowth of the wrong kind of bacteria in the vagina. Ear infections are often caused by the overgrowth of bacteria after water or soap get into the ear canal, disrupting the pH. Rather than antibiotics, GPs will often recommend slightly acidic eardrops, which return the pH in the direction preferred by the beneficial bacteria, allowing them to re-establish a healthy balance. As our understanding of the body's microbial populations develops, it is likely that more illnesses and infections that we currently treat with antibiotics will instead be administered with a dose of the right species of beneficial bacteria.

The gut microbiome is the population of microorganisms (bacteria, yeasts, fungi, archaea and viruses) that colonise the colon. Nowhere else on Earth is as densely populated with microbes as the human colon. But they are not just squatters hitching an easy ride. In return for a warm, moist place to live and a regular supply of the right foods, they more than pay us back. In fact, it is generally thought that humans and the microbes that colonise our guts evolved together in a mutually beneficial alliance based largely on a single nutrient: fibre.

Fibre

Actually, technically, fibre is not a single nutrient but a class of carbohydrates with a complex structure. This complexity means that we do not have the enzymes required to split the glucose molecules apart as we can with simpler sugars (see chapter 00). So fibre passes through our stomach and small intestine intact, where it then reaches the gut.

The UK's daily fibre intake recommendations are:

- Age 2–5 years: 15g a day.
- Age 5–11 years: 20g a day.
- Age 11–16 years: 25g a day.
- Age 16–18 years: 30g a day.
- Age 18 years and over: 30g a day.

For reference, here are the fibre contents of some common foods:

Food	Fibre per 100g
White rice, cooked	0.8
Brown rice, cooked	3
White bread	2.5
Wholewheat bread	6.9
Rye bread	9
White pasta	0.8
Wholewheat pasta	9.5
Cornflakes	3
Bran flakes	17

According to the most recent National Diet and Nutrition Survey the mean average intake of fibre was below recommended levels in every age group. Only 9 per cent of UK adults aged 19–64 consumed enough fibre. These very low dietary intakes are likely to be contributing to the rise in bowel cancer rates in younger people. And, I suggest, to poorer population brain and mental health.

The many species of bacteria in the human gut are specialised to break down fibre and, when they do, they produce a range of substances and effects important for host (us!) health. These by-products include short-chain fatty acids, B vitamins, vitamin K and neurotransmitters like serotonin, dopamine and acetylcholine. While these gut-derived neurotransmitters do not cross the blood-brain barrier, studies show that they both have an effect on the 500 million nerves of the enteric (gut) nervous system and communicate with the brain via the vagus nerve.

Short-Chain Fatty Acids

You are by now well acquainted with the long-chain fatty acids. Allow me to introduce the short-chain fatty acids (SCFAs). Produced by the microbial fermentation of fibre, the main SCFAs for our purposes are acetic acid (acetate), propionic acid (propionate) and butyric acid (butyrate). And they are *fascinating*. Here's a quick overview of some of their actions in the body:

- **Gut-barrier protection** – Butyrate is produced by *Clostridium*, *Eubacterium* and *Butyrivibrio* when they ferment resistant starches (found in foods like wholegrains, beans, legumes and cooked and cooled carbohydrates) and fructo-oligosaccharides (FOS) (bananas, onions and asparagus), and it is the main energy source of the epithelial cells that line the colon. Low fibre intake, and therefore low production of SCFAs, leads to intestinal permeability and increased inflammation in the gut. We have evidence that the same thing is happening in the brain.
- **Blood-brain barrier integrity** (see chapter 13).
- **Anti-inflammatory** – Butyrate turns on anti-inflammatory cytokines and can dampen inflammation in the gut, and also in the brain.
- **Neuroprotection** – Studies on cells and in animals show that treatment with butyrate can protect against oxidative stress and neuronal cell death. Some researchers hypothesise that gut-derived butyrate from a fibre-rich diet could provide an alternative energy source for the AD brain, which struggles to take up enough glucose for its needs.
- **Gene expression** – As I mentioned earlier our genes can be switched on or off, turned up or turned down depending on our experience with the world, and food is a key modulator of gene activity. The SCFAs produced by some strains of gut microbes affect gene expression. This could be one way in which psychological vulnerability is transmitted from parent to child.
- **Mood stabiliser** – A small pilot study looked at the association between mood, gut symptoms and ratios of SCFAs. They found that people with poorer mood and worse gut symptoms had lower levels of butyrate and propionate.

This evidence suggests that a high-fibre diet is neuroprotective, helping to support the survival of brain cells and prevent neurodegeneration. One of the big pitfalls for your brain when it comes to UPFs is the lack of fibre. The fibre- and vitamin-rich bran part of cereal grains tends to be higher in oils that can oxidise and spoil. So they are removed to extend shelf life.

The NHS website provides an example menu for an adult to meet the fibre intake recommendations (see below).

Breakfast

Two thick slices of wholemeal toasted bread (6.6g of fibre) topped with one sliced banana (1.4g) and a small glass (150ml) of fruit juice (1.2g) will give you around 9.2g of fibre.

Lunch

A baked jacket potato with the skin on (4.7g) with around half a can (about a 200g portion) of reduced-sugar and reduced-salt baked beans in tomato sauce (9.8g) followed by an apple (1.2g) will give you around 15.7g of fibre.

Dinner

Mixed vegetable tomato-based curry cooked with onion and spices (6.6g) with boiled wholegrain rice (2.7g) followed by a lower-fat fruit yoghurt (0.4g) will give you around 9.7g of fibre.

Snack

A small handful of nuts (30g), such as almonds, can have around 3.8g of fibre.

Total:

Around 38g of fibre.

Did you notice that the foods listed are predominantly un- or minimally processed? These have the fibres intact. Over 50 per cent of the UK adult diet is in the form of ultra-processed foods, which have typically had their fibre removed. It is incredibly difficult to achieve the recommended intake with this level of UPF consumption without supplementing with fibre directly.

So are fibre supplements the solution?

The food industry has noted the rise in both the research on the gut microbiome and the public appetite for higher-fibre foods and started to provide fibre-enriched UPFs. The fibre added to UPFs typically comes in the form of inulin, a soluble fibre that has been shown to support beneficial gut bacteria. This, in itself, is no bad thing. However, though there is still much to learn about what it means to have a 'healthy gut', the available data suggests that a diverse intake of fibres from a range of plant sources is the best way to support the gut microbiome. In the context of our currently very low population intake of fibre, supplements are definitely better than nothing, but they are not as good as what could be achieved from improved diet quality.

Beyond fibre, your gut microbiome benefits from a diverse range of plant foods, and a well-fed gut microbiome is associated with improved mood regulation. While there are 400,000 edible plants on the planet, we eat just a tiny fraction of these, around 200. Recent research suggests aiming for 30 different plant foods per week. This might sound daunting, but know that fruits, vegetables, nuts, seeds, beans, wholegrains, herbs and spices all count as plant foods. And yet more than half of our calories come from just three plants: corn, rice and wheat. Clearly there is some work to do.

Probiotics

Another gut-based intervention for mental health involves the introduction of commensal bacteria in the form of a probiotic supplement.

A study of depressed people compared the effect of supplementation with prebiotic fibre, probiotics or placebos for eight weeks. The probiotic led to a more significant decrease in depression. What was interesting about this study was that they also looked at the ratio of a substance called kynurenine to tryptophan. Tryptophan is an amino acid, a portion of a protein, and the building block of serotonin, the neurotransmitter that plays a role in mood regulation. When we are stressed or ill cytokines can trigger a cascade of reactions that pull tryptophan away from the production of serotonin and push it towards the kynurenine pathway. There are two major problems with this: (1) This leaves you with less serotonin to do its mood management job. (2) Kynurenine and other compounds produced on that pathway are neurotoxic. However, gut bacteria can reduce the activity of enzymes that push tryptophan down the kynurenine path and this is what they observed in this study; the participants taking the probiotics had a more favourable balance of kynurenine to tryptophan and less depression.

In a double-blind randomised controlled trial published in 2022 people with current symptoms of clinical depression took a commercially available multi-strain probiotic supplement or placebo for 31 days alongside their usual treatment. When they assessed the participants' gut microbiomes, they found an increase in the strain of bacteria called *Lactobacillus*. This rise was associated with a significantly larger decrease in depressive symptoms compared to the placebo group (who also improved). The researchers also scanned the brains of the participants and found that the probiotic group had increased grey matter (cell bodies that process information) volume more than the placebo group, and decreased activation in a part of the brain involved in emotional processing. The changes were seen in a part of the brain associated with the processing of visual information. These effects were most pronounced in the people with the highest compliance, indicating that consistency is crucial to accrue the benefit of an intervention like this.

On the flip side, evidence is growing that antibiotics increase the risk of sadness and depression. Antibiotics are prescribed to treat specific infections but, if they are taken orally, their effects are general, killing bacteria throughout the body, including the beneficial bacteria in the colon. A study of a million children born in Finland between 1996 and 2012 found an increased risk of ADHD, mood, anxiety and emotional disorders if those children had been exposed to antibiotics either through their mother's body during pregnancy or directly before the age of two. They were also more likely to be on antidepressants. A separate study of 871 mothers and their children conducted in New Zealand also found a similar association: antibiotic use in the first year of life was significantly linked to more parent- and teacher-rated ADHD symptoms and higher depression scores at age 11. And the story is the same for adults. When looking at the mental health of over a million Danes, and the same number of Brits, antibiotic use was associated with increased depression risk.

Taking care of our gut microbiota is a key but underappreciated feature of protecting our mental health. This means both feeding them well with a plentiful supply of varied types of fibre and limiting our exposure to antibiotics. Unfortunately, our high intake of UPFs means that hardly anyone is providing their microbiome with sufficient fibre for it to do its many important jobs protecting our gut lining, modulating inflammation and protecting BBB integrity.

Stressed Microbes

Another way that the microbiome can talk to and influence the brain is through our old friend, the stress-energy hormone cortisol.

Animal studies show that early life stress shapes the gut microbiome and is associated with increased inflammatory markers, with these changes persisting into adulthood.

A first-of-its-kind study published in 2019 looked at the relationship between early life stress, the microbiome and inflammation during pregnancy in humans. Women who were between 20 and 26 weeks pregnant were recruited. They completed a ten-item questionnaire designed to identify the number of adverse childhood experiences (ACEs – see the box on the next page) they had experienced. The questionnaire had a very simple 'yes/no' format with questions like: 'Did a parent or other adult in the household often . . . swear at you, insult you, put you down, or humiliate you? Or act in a way that made you afraid that you might be physically hurt?'

A 'yes' response was given a score of 1, a 'no' scored 0. Scores above 2 have, in previous research, been linked to a dysregulated stress response and increased risk of premature delivery. So in this study a score of 2 or more was considered high. The women also provided a stool sample for analysis of their gut microbiome and provided details of their diet. Then they were invited into the lab to participate in a test of social stress. Imagine doing mental arithmetic in front of an audience. Yep, that kind of stress. Blood samples were taken before and after to assess their cortisol levels. They found that greater childhood stress was linked to altered gut microbiome and a dysregulated stress response. Fascinatingly, higher intake of omega-3 DHA in the high ACE women dampened their stress-induced inflammation.

In a more recent study using the same social stress test, 138 middle-aged people took either a placebo, 1.25g of omega-3 per day or 2.5g of omega-3 per day. Both the supplement groups had significantly lower stress and inflammation compared to the placebo group. They also had improved markers of cellular repair, indicative of slower cellular aging.

These results make the point that, while good food is not a panacea for mental health, improved nutrition is an accessible way to mitigate the impact of life events, a shock absorber for the earthquakes we cannot avoid.

ADVERSE CHILDHOOD EXPERIENCES

While the exact mechanisms for depression are still being worked out, we do know that certain experiences, particularly in early life, increase a person's chance of developing depression in adulthood. These ACEs include:

- Physical abuse
- Sexual abuse
- Emotional abuse
- Abandonment
- Neglect

- Living with someone who abused drugs and/or alcohol
- Experiencing domestic violence
- Having an incarcerated parent
- Living with someone with serious mental illness
- Losing a parent through divorce
- The death of a parent

ACEs seem to programme a dysregulated stress response. People with an ACE history have higher baseline levels of pro-inflammatory cytokines C-reactive protein, IL6, nuclear factor κB and tumor necrosis factor (TNF-α). That is, they are predisposed to low-grade chronic inflammation. The downstream consequences of chronically elevated inflammation are likely to play a major role in the increased depression risk.

Whether it is through its metabolites such as short-chain fatty acids and neurotransmitters, protection of the gut lining, regulation of the immune system, modulation of the stress (hypothalamic-pituitary-adrenal (HPA) axis, or supporting BBB integrity, the gut microbiome plays a key role in brain structure and function. No wonder we call them 'friendly' bacteria! The evidence we have so far tells us that the best way to support the microbiome is through the consumption of adequate and diverse sources of fibre. Our reliance on ultra-processed foods makes this impossible.

A TALE OF TWO BRAINS

Neither Anya nor Mia really knew anything about the gut microbiome until influencers they followed on Instagram started talking about it.

Anya was pretty happy that she was eating a good range of vegetables and fruits. She ate hummus regularly but realised she could eat a broader range of beans. She thought it might be a good idea to stop buying hummus and start making her own with mixed beans.

She swapped her porridge oats for mixed grains and switched to a seeded wholegrain bread. Regular consumption of fibre may help to reduce the production of pro-Alzheimer's proteins, so by making these changes Anya is supporting her long-term brain health. Higher-fibre foods also help to maintain steady blood sugar levels, which, as discussed, is beneficial too.

Having grown up eating the more refined versions, Mia didn't really like the taste of wholemeal bread or brown pasta, but she did her best, choosing the 'half and half' brands, such as white bread with added fibre. Unfortunately, like most people in the UK, she did not meet the fibre recommendations. Knowing how important fibre-derived SCFAs are we can assume that her gut and blood-brain barrier are not as well protected as they could be. Since pro-inflammatory gut microbes are kept in check by fibre consumption, she may have higher proportions of these harmful species.

CHAPTER 9

ALCOHOL

OKAY, AFTER ALL of that, maybe you're thinking, 'I need a drink!' So let's talk about alcohol and its effects on the brain. First, though, there are a few controversies about the substance so I want to be clear on one thing: alcohol (ethanol) is a neurotoxin. That means it damages and kills brain cells. Furthermore, alongside asbestos, tobacco and radiation it is classified as a group 1 carcinogen. I wanted to get that out of the way so there is no confusion. In the UK we have normalised alcohol consumption so much that people feel they need to have a valid reason *not* to consume it. We don't treat any other drug in this way. And we should be clear on that too: alcohol is a drug with potent psychoactive effects. So, if you do not drink alcohol, you should not feel in any way awkward about it, and you can probably skip this entire chapter. Everyone else, I think it is important that you understand more about alcohol and your brain so you can make informed decisions about your consumption.

The product of alcohol metabolism in the body is acetaldehyde, which, aside from being the main culprit behind hangovers, increases neuroinflammation (harmful inflammation in the brain), oxidative stress and excitotoxicity (nerve damage from excessive activation) events in the brain. The harms of alcohol consumption are associated with the frequency, quantity and duration of drinking. And we have evidence of harms from early in life.

Alcohol During Pregnancy

For a time, up until around the 1960s, it was believed that Guinness was a good source of iron. Consequently it was prescribed to pregnant women (who have an increased iron need) to help them stave off anaemia. For the record, it is unclear where this spurious claim originated, since Guinness contains essentially no iron at all. This advice almost certainly did more harm than good. In May 2007 the Department of Health updated the recommendations on alcohol consumption during pregnancy. Until that point women had been advised that it was safe to drink small, infrequent amounts of alcohol throughout pregnancy, not more than 'one to two units of alcohol once or twice a week'. The new guidance advises women to avoid alcohol completely. But apparently there is still some confusion. As recently as 2021 parenting websites were still answering the question 'Can you drink Guinness when pregnant?' and many people still believe it is a good source of iron.

The most recent comprehensive UK data on pregnancy and alcohol consumption comes from the Infant Feeding Survey published in 2010. It found that 40 per cent of women drank during pregnancy, the vast majority drank two or fewer units of alcohol per week. Older, wealthier, white women were the most likely to drink during their pregnancy. Although rates of drinking during pregnancy are dropping both in the UK and around the world, the UK still ranks fourth highest in the world for rates of drinking during pregnancy according to a review published in 2017, which also estimated that one in every 67 women who drinks alcohol during her pregnancy will give birth to a child with foetal alcohol syndrome. A smaller, prospective cohort study of 1,303 UK women found that 79 per cent, 63 per cent and 49 per cent consumed alcohol during trimesters 1, 2 and 3, respectively, a figure substantially higher than the Infant Feeding Survey. The researchers remark that even this could be an underestimate because people very commonly underreport their alcohol intake. In this study, consuming more than two units per week during the first and second trimesters was associated with increased risk of low birth weight, and an elevated risk of preterm birth if the mother drank during trimester 1.

They conclude:

Pregnant women and women planning to become pregnant should be advised to abstain from drinking, as even those women who adhered to the UK guidelines of 1–2 units once or twice a week in the first trimester were at risk of having babies with reduced birth weight and born preterm when compared to mothers who abstained from alcohol.

Ethanol easily crosses the placenta, entering foetal circulation at the same blood alcohol concentration as the mother's. However, the foetus's underdeveloped liver cannot process the alcohol efficiently, meaning that it remains in the body for a long time, increasing the opportunity to cause harm to fragile developing tissues. Alcohol is a teratogen, which means that it can cause birth defects in the developing foetus. Foetal alcohol spectrum disorder (FASD) is the umbrella term for a range of lifelong physical and neurological conditions affecting children born to mothers who drink during pregnancy. They include behavioural problems, difficulties regulating emotions and poorer impulse control, as well as learning difficulties and impaired cognition.

Of course, we cannot get pregnant women drunk in order to see what happens to their babies, so the best evidence of the effects of alcohol consumption during pregnancy is a combination of animal studies and observational human data.

We do not actually have prevalence data for FASD in the UK. However, although full foetal alcohol syndrome is rare, it is the leading cause of non-genetic learning difficulties in the world, and since the European region is the world leader in pregnancy alcohol consumption, and two in five UK women (at last count) consumed alcohol during pregnancy, it is a message that is relevant to the population.

Later Harms

The NHS uses two definitions for measuring alcohol-related hospital admissions. The narrow definition relates to instances where only the primary diagnosis relates to alcohol. The broad definition allows for either the first or second diagnosis to be alcohol-related. According to official NHS statistics, under the narrow definition, there were 358,000 UK hospital admissions where the main reason cited was alcohol in 2018–19. This was up 6 per cent on the 2017–18 figures and nearly 20 per cent higher than 2008–09. Under the broad definition, there were 976,425 alcohol-related hospital admissions.

In my experience, if someone is concerned about their alcohol consumption it is either due to the associated weight gain or the behavioural consequences. Patients will complain of not being able to lose weight and will be shocked when I tell them that the beers they drink in the evening to 'wind down' work out to 84 units of alcohol, contributing over 4,700 calories to their weekly consumption. Or they will not like the angry, nihilistic person they become when they drink too much. Or simply that they cannot control their consumption. A friend of mine started going to Alcoholics Anonymous meetings not because she had hit 'rock bottom', but because she realised that she couldn't stop at just one glass of wine. However, what most people are generally not thinking about is the potential impact of their drinking on their long-term brain health and, to be honest, they probably should.

When it comes to adult intake, there continues to be some controversy over the role of low to moderate alcohol consumption on brain health. Observational Mediterranean diet studies often conclude that consumption of a small amount of red wine might confer some benefits and several studies have indicated a 'J-shaped curve' in terms of alcohol's harms. Here non-drinkers seem to have higher illness rates than moderate drinkers, with the risks increasing again with higher alcohol intake.

The difficulty with assessing the health effects of alcohol consumption is making sense of the health status of non-drinkers. On the one hand you might have someone who abstains for religious reasons. Or an uber-health-conscious athlete who can't risk impairing their performance. But many people who avoid alcohol do so because they are in recovery from addiction, in which case their body and brain health might already be compromised, the so-called 'sick quitters'.

Alcohol Consumption and General Health

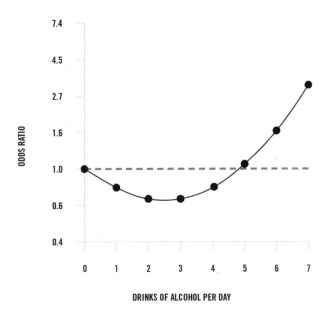

DRINKS OF ALCOHOL PER DAY

— — — Dashed line indicates average alcohol consumption

Alternatively, people often give up alcohol when they are actively trying to lose weight or improve their health in some other way. All of which is to say that, for many, abstinence from alcohol could be a marker of some other health risk.

The other difficulty is in distinguishing red wine consumption from other features of the Mediterranean lifestyle. For example, when people drink moderately it tends to be in the context of a meal, often with other people. Nutritious food and good social connections are known protective factors for brain health, meaning that the identified benefits could be more to do with the food and the company than the wine.

That said, there is some mechanistic (theoretical) evidence to suggest that small amounts of alcohol, particularly red wine, could be beneficial to the brain. Researchers cite the known brain benefits of polyphenols, beneficial plant compounds, many of which give fruits

and vegetables their bright or deep colour. In studies in which participants are given a polyphenol-rich drink compared to placebo, we see
very rapid (within two hours) improvements in brain blood flow and
associated cognitive enhancement. *In vitro* studies have shown that
some classes of polyphenols inhibit the aggregation of beta-amyloid,
the sticky protein that is a hallmark of Alzheimer's disease, providing a
plausible mechanism for why berries and other polyphenol-rich foods
seems to be neuroprotective. For this reason it is assumed that, if there
is something in red wine that is conferring neurological benefits, it is
the 'red' rather than the wine. It is conceivable that at low to moderate
levels of consumption the benefits of the polyphenols in red wine *just
about* outweigh the risks of the ethanol. However, this remains a highly
controversial area of nutrition research. Most people who drink alcohol would probably benefit from cutting back. If you do not drink, the
advice is not to start simply for the potential brain health benefits. Of
course, you can enjoy alcohol-free polyphenols by consuming berries
and other brightly coloured fruits and vegetables, dark chocolate, tea
and coffee.

Binge Drinking

The UK government defines binge drinking as: males who exceed
eight units on their heaviest drinking day (around four pints of normal-
strength beer or three-quarters of a bottle of wine) and females who
exceed six units on their heaviest drinking day (around three pints of
normal-strength beer or two large glasses of wine). Young people
(aged 16–24) are currently the group least likely to consume alcohol
overall. However, when they do, they are more likely than other age
groups to drink in a binge-type pattern, drinking heavily on Friday and
Saturday nights. This is of particular concern because the brain is still
maturing during this period of life. Alcohol can inhibit neurogenesis, a
key feature of neuroplasticity, which could potentially lead to long-
term structural and functional changes in the adolescent brain.

Midlife alcohol consumption is one of the modifiable risk factors for
dementia listed by the *Lancet* Commission (see page 199). Worryingly,

this age group is the most likely to drink at higher risk levels. At the same time teetotalism has dropped in this group, driven largely by fewer women in this age group reporting that they do not drink. The number of alcohol-related hospital admissions rises with age, peaking in 55- to 64-year-olds, before falling. While middle-aged men are still more likely to drink than middle-aged women, the fact that women have twice the Alzheimer's risk of men makes this a potential concern.

A SMALL GLASS OF WINE

It is worth being clear about what we mean when we say a 'small glass of wine', as the volumes described in the research literature differ somewhat from what might be considered a small serving at home or at a bar.

In the UK the law dictates the standard serving size of alcohol when purchased for on-site consumption, i.e. in a pub, bar or restaurant. For wine the 'specified quantities' are 125ml and 175ml (and multiples thereof). So a small glass of wine is typically 125ml.

However, you may be surprised (and dismayed) to learn that, depending on the study, the recommended limit is around 75–150ml of red wine per day for women and 200–300ml for men.

In addition, wine that is enjoyed with food tends to be consumed more slowly, lowering the rate of absorption and potentially reducing the alcohol processing burden on the liver.

While the scientists work on clearing up the confusion regarding zero vs low alcohol intake, what is not debated is the negative consequences of high and binge-type alcohol consumption on brain structure and function. Heavy alcohol consumption is one of the key modifiable risk factors for young-onset dementia (YOD), which is dementia that emerges before the age of 65. In one study of over 57,000 instances of YOD, 39 per cent of cases were identified as alcohol-related brain damage. In older people around 10–24 per cent of dementia cases are understood to be alcohol-associated.

Wernicke-Korsakoff Syndrome

Thiamine (aka vitamin B1), which we met in chapter 6 during our discussion of diabetes, is found in trout, pork, wholegrains, peas and beans, nuts and liver, and it is often added to fortified breakfast cereals. The body is only able to store small amounts so daily dietary intake is required.

In 1884 a Japanese doctor noted that sailors who were at sea for prolonged periods with only white rice to eat became sick, and many died. If, on their return, the sick sailors were fed a diet of wholegrains, beans and some meat they recovered. Later, Dutch scientists noticed that chickens fed only white rice developed paralysis of the legs, but those fed brown rice did not. However, it took a few more years for them to deduce that there was some 'protective substance' (thiamine) in the rice husks.

Thiamine is an essential co-factor for enzymes in the brain required for glucose metabolism. As mentioned previously, the brain has a huge glucose demand relative to its size, suggesting that the brain will be particularly sensitive to thiamine availability.

Beriberi is a condition caused by thiamine deficiency. There are two main types: wet, which affects the cardiovascular system with symptoms such as increased heart rate; and dry, which affects the nervous system. The impairments to the nervous system in dry beriberi include peripheral neuropathy (numbness in the hands and feet), difficulty walking or moving the legs (like the aforementioned chickens) and pain. The effects on the central nervous system include confusion and difficulty generating speech.

Alcohol reduces the absorption of thiamine, which means that excessive and chronic alcohol consumption, especially in the context of a poor diet, can create thiamine deficiency and the development of Wernicke-Korsakoff syndrome (WKS). WKS is an extreme form of thiamine deficiency, which involves the development of areas of brain damage, involuntary movements of the eyes and body, amnesia and other memory problems. Alcohol also depletes the body's stores of omega-3 fats, creating a potent brain assault.

Researchers have highlighted the similarities between WKS and Alzheimer's disease. For example, thiamine deficiency results in the same magnitude of impaired glucose metabolism as is seen in AD. Poor glucose metabolism in WKS is restored with thiamine treatment. Similarly, thiamine-dependent enzymes are reduced in AD brains. Both thiamine deficiency syndromes (like beriberi and WKS) and AD involve memory impairments. While this does not mean that AD could be treated with thiamine, it could suggest a role of thiamine dysfunction in the progression of Alzheimer's. In fact, some suggest that long-term thiamine deficiency may be an early trigger for the later development of AD.

ALCOHOL, ANXIETY AND DEPRESSION

Not only do hangovers increase the likelihood of experiencing anxiety, but it is estimated that around 20–27 per cent of people with social anxiety disorder have problematic drinking behaviours and rely on alcohol to provide them with 'Dutch courage' and confidence in social situations.

Economists and social scientists have shown that social inequality increases anxiety-driven status threat. The lower down one feels on the social ladder, the more anxious we are about being looked down on and judged as inferior. For many this will increase the reliance on alcohol as a solution to their 'confidence issues', demonstrating another mechanism through which social gradients drive health inequality and place a disproportionate health burden on disadvantaged groups.

The relationship between alcohol consumption and depressive symptoms is well established and bidirectional: drinking increases depressive moods and people often turn to alcohol to temporarily relieve depression or numb their feelings.

So What Can We Do?

About 20 per cent of consumed alcohol is absorbed in the stomach with the remainder absorbed in the small intestine. Some of the contradictory findings on the role of alcohol consumption on brain health and function may be related to the way in which it is consumed. As mentioned, when alcohol is consumed as part of the Mediterranean diet, it typically accompanies a meal. The presence of macronutrients (proteins, carbohydrates and fats) in the stomach can slow the transit and absorption of alcohol in the gastrointestinal tract. This can reduce the burden on the liver, whose job it is to break down alcohol. So, if you drink, the advice is to try to do so with meals and keep within the recommended limits.

The good news is that the overall trend for alcohol consumption in the UK seems to be going down. More people than ever are staying within the recommended levels and many are either abstaining or ensuring that they are taking regular breaks.

On a population level, minimum unit pricing is an effective strategy. Minimum unit pricing is a system that sets a fixed base price, under which an alcohol product is not permitted to be sold. The World Health Organization estimates that this system could reduce the gap in alcohol-attributable deaths between high- and low-income groups by 30 per cent. With the rising number of alcohol-related hospital admissions, this would be something worth considering. Similar strategies have been successful in shifting population behaviour in the recent past, most notably the levy on plastic bags (see page 250). Currently, though, the cost of alcohol in the UK is going down. And since we have a government known for its fondness for cheese and wine work gatherings, it seems unlikely that any restrictions or taxes that might reduce the availability or affordability of alcohol will be popular. At the very least, the associations between moderate to heavy alcohol consumption and cognitive impairment and dementia should be made clear, as part of a public brain health campaign, so that people who decide to drink can make an informed choice.

A TALE OF TWO BRAINS

Anya's mother and *yiayia* would often have a small glass of red wine with dinner. Though her mother would drink a little more at family parties, Anya couldn't remember ever seeing her drunk. Growing up, Anya was allowed a tiny bit of diluted wine at her mother's discretion on family occasions. When she reached adolescence, her association with alcohol was as a beverage consumed with a meal in relatively small amounts. She drank a bit more as a teenager but she noticed that alcohol never really seemed as exciting to her as it did to her friends.

As a teenager and young adult Mia got into the habit of drinking pretty heavily on Friday or Saturday nights (often both). During the summer it was common to go drinking after work, making the most of the sunny weather. She learned to keep her Sundays free as a recovery from Friday and Saturday nights.

Excessive alcohol consumption is a significant cause of brain damage and dementia. While it is hard to know for sure the exact effects on her brain, we know that alcohol consumption is the largest modifiable contributing factor to brain shrinkage and recent studies suggest that any amount of alcohol has a negative effect on the brain. Given the other nutrition factors that her brain is contending with (low fibre, omega-3s and B vitamins; high sugar) Mia's brain will be less able to withstand the harms of alcohol.

CHAPTER 10

FOOD, SCHOOL EXCLUSION AND THE CYCLE OF POVERTY

For want of a nail the shoe was lost.
For want of a shoe the horse was lost.
For want of a horse the rider was lost.
For want of a rider the battle was lost.
For want of a battle the kingdom was lost.
And all for the want of a horseshoe nail.

THIS PROVERB ILLUSTRATES how imperceptible errors or omissions early on in a trajectory can have outsize downstream consequences. We've covered a lot of ground over the last nine chapters, in terms of exploring nutrition's contribution to our brain development and behaviour. Maternal DHA during pregnancy affects infant brain size, neuronal connectivity and, potentially, IQ. We have seen in the case of choline that a single nutrient can significantly improve attention in children years later, and that attention is a predictor of maths and language ability. In turn, the advantages of prenatal and early life nutritional sufficiency may contribute to greater academic success, the greater self-confidence that comes with that and the positive life outcomes associated with these features. Better maternal nutrition sets children on a positive trajectory. But what about the flip side? What might be the downstream consequences of nutritional deficiency in childhood and adolescence? Is there evidence that nutritional status in childhood affects school performance, behaviour or mental health?

Hunger, Malnutrition and Children's Behaviour

Children lack the experience and vocabulary to comprehend, communicate and manage their emotional experiences. More often, their psychological distress is expressed in their behaviour. Psychologists typically categorise these behaviours as 'internalising' or 'externalising'. Internalising behaviours include nervousness, sadness, withdrawal, difficulty concentrating, not talking, sleep disturbance and somatic complaints such as stomach aches and headaches. Internalising behaviours are common in depressed children. By contrast, externalising behaviours include aggression, impulsivity, defiance, bullying, vandalism and other destructive acts. As with internalising behaviours, externalising behaviours are an indicator of a child who is struggling in some way but they are also a significant risk factor for juvenile delinquency, violence and adult crime. Interestingly, poor nutrition in early life can affect both behaviour patterns. For example, higher levels of DHA recorded at birth were linked to fewer internalising behaviour problems at age seven.

Poor nutrition in childhood can influence brain development in such a way as to increase the likelihood of later violence and aggression. In a longitudinal study of children born on the island of Mauritius, there was a dose-response relationship between malnutrition as assessed at age three and aggression at age eight, externalising behaviour at 11 and conduct disorder at 17. Similarly, Barbadian adolescents who experienced malnutrition in early life were more likely to report conduct disorder than their well-nourished peers. In explaining the results, the researchers hypothesised that nutritional deficiencies experienced during the critical period of brain development impaired brain formation and cognition, predisposing children to greater violence. To put it simply: inadequate nutrition impairs brain development and cognition (thinking, reasoning, planning, emotion regulation), inclining the individual to externalising behaviours including violence and aggression. And, according to government data published in 2022, this kind of disruptive behaviour is the main reason for children being excluded from school. So, is there a link between poor nutrition and school exclusion?

School exclusion

Children who are in receipt of free school meals are four times more likely to be excluded from school than children from wealthier households. Some of that difference is attributable to other factors associated with lower household income such as greater parental stress, which can negatively affect parenting style and subsequent child behaviour. But what do we know about the contribution of nutrition and hunger itself on children's academic and life outcomes?

To start answering that question, it's worth thinking about why hunger is such as big deal in the first place. Most humans in wealthy nations carry sufficient body fat to provide several weeks' worth of calories. You would imagine then that a moment of transient hunger would be shrugged off as little more than a mild inconvenience. However, we have to remember: (1) our brains are extraordinarily hungry (and important organs); and (2) evolution has programmed our brain-bodies to be exquisitely sensitive to indicators of reduced food availability and famine. In short, when your brain-body recognises that energy stores are being tapped into, brain-body chemistry shifts in a way that affects mood and behaviour.

The first evolutionary tool is discomfort, the effect of which is clearly observable in babies. When babies are hungry, they experience an internal state of unpleasantness that they communicate through crying. As children grow and develop greater awareness and descriptive vocabulary, they are able to give a name to these sensations and ask for their needs to be met: 'I'm hungry. Can I have a snack?' However, we might recognise these feelings of hunger only after they have reached a certain threshold; for example, a 2 or a 3 on a scale of 1–10, where 1 is ravenous and 10 is stuffed to the gills. But the body-brain will be 'aware' of our movement down the scale from the moment of the last bite of the previous meal.

The next tool is cortisol. As blood glucose begins to drop cortisol begins to rise. One of the side effects of cortisol is the production of a state of agitation that might be subjectively experienced as anything from restlessness to aggression. For several years the term 'hanger' has been used colloquially to describe feelings of irritability and anger associated with hunger. But there is now science to back up this phenomenon. Firstly, increased aggression is also commonly seen in hungry animals, including flies and goats, compared to their well-fed counterparts. This increased aggression and impulsivity is understood to be an evolutionary adaptation: when resources are scarce it is the bolder, more aggressive individual that is more likely to secure food, compared to the more timid members of the group. But what about us?

A recent study asked 64 European adults (average age 30) to provide repeated measures of their hunger, irritability and anger on a scale of 1–100. After 21 days the researchers analysed the results and found associations between the three parameters. What was remarkable was the extent of the association. Hunger accounted for 52 per cent of the variance in irritability and 48 per cent for anger. There were also associated declines in feelings of pleasure (see Valence, page 191). In short, hunger makes us feel rotten, and predisposes us to more aggressive feelings, all operating below our conscious awareness. Additionally, hunger has consistently been associated with poorer self-control.

Food insecurity and hunger are also sources of *toxic stress*; stress from which there is inadequate time and opportunity to recover. This leaves the child in a state of prolonged activation of the stress system. The brain is not adapted to tolerate prolonged stress of this kind. Chronic corticosteroid secretion is corrosive to the prefrontal cortex, hippocampus and other cortisol-receptor-dense areas; it causes brain cells to shrink and eventually die. In this sense the brain is being attacked from both sides – malnutrition and the physical stress of hunger limit brain development and undermine psychological health. Hungry children have twice the parent-rated anxiety as their non-hungry classmates and suffer increased irritability and poorer self-regulation (in other words, they are less well behaved).

Putting this together we see a pattern emerging. Firstly, strong intersecting relationships between hunger, stress and mood. More specifically, hunger is associated with increased irritability, aggression and less impulse control. When we are hungry we are more prone to act first and think second. And this is what we see in children. Hungry children are more prone to irritability, low mood and impulsivity. These affective states not only impair a child's ability to concentrate on schoolwork, but also lower their capacity to engage with friends and can contribute to disruptive behaviour. Furthermore, children find it more difficult to manage their emotions, meaning it is harder for them (compared to adults) to suppress negative emotional states and the associated behaviours.

A poll of primary-school teachers in England conducted in August 2022 found that hungry children in their schools showed signs of being excessively tired, easily distracted from their schoolwork, anxious and disruptive in class. To learn more about the realities and consequences of child hunger in schools I spoke to Carmel McConnell MBE, founder of the charity Magic Breakfast, which aims 'to end hunger as a barrier to education in UK schools through the provision of healthy breakfasts to children living with food insecurity'. I asked her what inspired her to start the charity. She explained that, at the time, she had been researching a book about social change:

> *It was back in 2000 . . . I got five headteachers together in Hackney and I said, 'For us in the city, across the business community, do you think that we're helping you to create a fairer as well as a richer society?' And they said, 'Every single person in my team, Carmel' – every headteacher said it – 'has to bring in food every single day just to be able to teach. If my teachers don't get food on the way in to give out to their kids in the morning you just cannot teach, and the most important lessons are taught in the morning. So, if we've got any chance at all of maths at ten o'clock they've got to bring in bananas, biscuits, because by half-nine, ten, the hands are up and, "Miss, I've got a tummy ache", or a child will be fainting.' I said, 'Really? Hang on. Breakfast is not expensive.*

Why aren't the parents giving their children breakfast before they come to school?' And they were saying, 'Look, Carmel, the parents are hungry themselves, they're in insecure work, their rent is half their wages ... for a lot of them they haven't got any money, they've run out of money, and so the only thing that they can adjust down – it's not their electricity, it's not their rent, it's their food bill. And so some of these kids are coming in from homes without food, and so they're in the bins in Tesco.'

And it was one of those moments. I just couldn't believe it. Here I am talking about lofty social purpose and business and blah blah and these teachers were telling me that there was just no way that they could even begin to do what they'd trained for unless they brought in food because the kids were so hungry. I was so upset. So I said, 'I know nothing about nutrition but I'm really happy to drop off some cereal and some food on Saturday mornings', as a thank you. But being geeky, being a technology person, I said, 'Can we do some kind of baseline? Can I see whether this is useful to you or not.' So [we looked at] punctuality and how many fights there were in first break. Within the first two weeks they had improved punctuality, really considerably, in all five schools and they had seen a drop of about 30 per cent of first-break fights.

Returning to the evidence that disruptive behaviours are the most common reason that children are excluded from school, and that children in receipt of free school meals are four times more likely to experience exclusion, this raises the very real possibility that there are children in the UK who are at increased risk of being kicked out of school simply because they are hungry. And the 'cost of living crisis' will increase the number of children in this devastating and unfair position. We have a situation where, on paper, families look like they can afford to pay for their children's school lunches but that assessment has not taken into account inflation, and the rise in fuel and energy prices. At the time of writing nearly a million children fall into this affordability gap.

MENTAL HEALTH IN SCHOOLS

There may be even more reason to focus on improving school nutrition. Large studies are finding null or even iatrogenic (where the treatments make things worse) effects of mental health interventions in schools. A large study of mindfulness, for example, found that the intervention did not reduce psychological distress in children, and for some made it worse, causing them to focus more on their negative feelings. Mental health treatments are best targeted at those most likely to benefit.

Given these disappointing results, improved nutrition – whether through supplementation or improved food quality – presents a low-risk, economical way of improving the poor mental health of children and young people, without the negative effects.

It seems to me that as well as the moral case (that feeding hungry children is just the decent thing to do) we also have a clinical and public health case for ensuring that no child goes hungry, particularly in a nation like the UK, which in 2020 was the fifth largest global economy according to data from World Bank. Yet, in the same year as it achieved this impressive chart position, and in the first six months of the Covid-19 pandemic when families on low incomes were hardest hit by the lockdown and job losses, the government voted against extending the provision of food vouchers that would support England's 1.4 million most disadvantaged children. The parliamentary motion, tabled by the Labour Party, to continue to provide vouchers worth £15 per week was voted down by the Conservatives. Some 322 Conservative Party members voted against it, including the then children's minister, Vicky Ford. This vote left children in England without this provision as both the Welsh and Scottish parliaments voted in favour of continuing.

The official line at the time was that the government was providing sufficient support to families through the welfare system but those on the ground paint a vastly different picture. A survey of primary-school teachers commissioned by the charity Chefs in Schools shows that:

- 83 per cent say that there are children who come to school hungry because their parents/guardians cannot afford enough food.
- 81 per cent say that the number of children coming to school hungry is increasing.
- 23 per cent see children who skip lunch due to poverty, while 79 per cent see children bring insufficient food to school for their packed lunch.
- 85 per cent agree that in their school there are children who are ineligible for free school meals who would benefit from receiving them.

Is it ignorance or arrogance that sees ministers dismiss the expertise of teachers and education professionals who work with children on a daily basis and can see both the inadequacy of provision and the impact of hunger on their wellbeing and school performance?

The vote against appears even more punitive (if not outright cruel) when contrasted with the ensuing scandal over the government's allocation of private sector contracts during this period. Extending the voucher scheme would have cost £157 million. In contrast, an investigation by the *Sunday Times* revealed that £1.5 billion worth of government money went to companies with links to the Conservative Party. 'None of the firms were prominent government suppliers before this year.' Contracts worth £18 billion were signed during the first six months of the Covid-19 crisis without a formal tendering process, with ongoing concerns about potential fraud and cronyism. They had enough money. They had enough money to give to their friends and donors. They *chose* not to spend it on ensuring vulnerable children had enough to eat.

At the same time expertly prepared meals in Parliament are subsidised by the taxpayer to the tune of £25 million (across three years). I am not necessarily against public servants enjoying a delicious and nutritious meal but there is more than a hint of hypocrisy in the notion that a wealthy, well-fed individual, who holds one of the most powerful positions in the country, should have their lunch subsidised by the taxpayer while there are children going hungry. And despite the Members' Dining Room ensuring 'the best regional and organic produce is at the heart of all our menus' some peers aren't even grateful about the provision. 'There are only so many smoked salmon or prawn and crayfish salads one can take week after week,' according to one complaint.

'It's Not the Government's Job to Feed Hungry Kids'

Yet, feeding hungry children can be a surprisingly controversial subject when it should, to my mind, be a staggeringly simple moral position: the need to protect vulnerable children. One of the arguments that was often raised during this time, at least on social media, against extending the benefit was that you would be inadvertently rewarding feckless parents. 'It's the job of the parent(s) to feed their own children. They should budget better.' Classist aspersions were thrown around with abandon. 'The parents shouldn't be spending all their money on booze and fags and bingo.' To be clear, many people went to great lengths to dispel the myth that food vouchers were being exchanged for beers and suchlike. Similarly, others have noted how rising fuel costs and inflation have contributed to the 'cost of living squeeze', which, you will recall, is a political euphemism for 'more children and their families will be pushed into poverty'.

But for me this isn't even close to the point.

Far from the tired stereotype of career benefit claimants who feel entitled to be taken care of by the state, many parents whose children are in receipt of free school meal vouchers are in work. Some 60 per cent of people in poverty in the UK live in a household where at least one person is working, and the rate is growing. They are the fabled 'hard-working families' that political speechwriters are so keen to woo. These are individuals who are doing all the right things and yet their incomes cannot cover the high cost of private rent in a housing market with insufficient social housing stock. Poverty researcher Dr Rod Hick explains that 'the private rented sector is associated with high housing costs, and elevated poverty rates, and a continued shift towards the private rented sector is likely to generate upward pressures on poverty rates in the UK'. So the notion that benefit claimants are just sitting around waiting for effortless money to arrive is incorrect and cruel.

But let's say, for the sake of argument, that the most disparaging characterisations of these parents and caretakers were correct. That rather than assiduously organising their budgets in order to try to eke out the money to pay for rent, electricity, gas, water, phone, TV licence, toiletries, transport, clothing and food, they blow it all on [insert your choice of egregious spending here] leaving their children without enough food to eat. Isn't that child *even more vulnerable* than the child whose parents are unable to feed them despite their best efforts? How, then, is denying that child access to food construed as a moral victory? Some people, intoxicated by the opportunity to exact righteous vengeance, to teach the parents a lesson, were willing to make children collateral damage to their ideals.

The evidence is clear that hunger and undernutrition in childhood increase antisocial behaviour, social exclusion, anxiety, depression, suicidal ideation and risk of school expulsion. Permitting children to go hungry because you are angry with their parents is not a moral victory.

The silver lining of this disappointing decision by British politicians is that the British public, despite our world-famous cynicism, were a beacon of decency and compassion for these children. The public's response to the government's failure of moral leadership still moves me to tears. Thousands of meals were provided as local restaurants and cafes, soup kitchens and faith congregations, community groups and individuals put together lunch packs for children to come and collect. Many went out of their way to make delivery or pick-up of these packs anonymous or discreet, being mindful of how poverty can unfairly engender feelings of shame in children and their parents. That so many people, most of whom had not experienced that kind of profound hunger or poverty themselves, were motivated to such generosity and altruism, particularly when those traits were not on display from the country's leadership, is something to be immensely proud of.

But we can't simply rely on public goodwill to plug the gaps in policy. I hope that these same thousands can be motivated to lobby their MPs to apply political pressure to advocate for policies that support vulnerable children and their families.

It is, of course, a great shame that we should have to. When private citizens, be they footballers, dinner ladies or celebrity chefs, have to do the work of the government, you know the system is failing.

Food and the Cycle of Poverty

Calorie for calorie, healthier foods are on average three times more expensive than less healthy, more processed foods, and if this trend continues (as it is predicted to) then healthier diets will simply become unaffordable for many. Already, wealthier women are more likely to adhere to a healthy diet during pregnancy. In studies that look at UPFD consumption in children, it is the children of poorer mothers who are more likely to eat industrially produced foods and more of them. Why is this? As well as being cheaper, they are quicker to prepare so use less energy. There is also a greater density of fast-food outlets and advertising in areas of deprivation compared to wealthier regions.

So, poorer people are priced out of healthier diets. What else do we know about the impact of social inequality on public health? The Indian caste system provides a powerful example of the strong relationship between social status, wealth and health. In India (and the Indian diaspora) the majority Hindu population is hierarchically organised into castes, which dictate someone's social position in a rigid and reinforced structure that is near impossible to escape.

The castes in descending order are Brahmins, Kshatriyas, Vaishyas and Shudras. People considered so lowly as not to have a class – Dalits or Scheduled Caste – are considered 'impure' or 'untouchable', and live under the constant threat of violence or exclusion. Caste membership is considered hereditary and signified by surname, making someone's social position instantly recognisable on introduction. Furthermore, individuals typically marry within their caste. This means that wide-scale discrimination severely limits the opportunities for social mobility and the outcome is that people in this group experience huge levels of health and economic disadvantage. In India a woman from a dominant caste lives 15 years longer than a Dalit woman. And in the UK? A reminder that, here, the poorest live with 19 additional years of ill health and die seven years sooner than the rich. But this differential was not created by millennia of faith-based discrimination. So how did we get here?

The Marmot review

The first Marmot review, a report into health inequalities in England, was commissioned in 2008 by the Labour Party. A few months after it was completed the Liberal Democrat–Conservative coalition government was in power. An updated report, published in February 2020, reviewing national health trends since 2010, showed that the health gap is widening between the wealthiest and most deprived parts of the country. The fall in life expectancy in women in the more deprived areas reverses what had been an upward trend for decades. If 'health is a good measure of social and economic progress' then our social and economic progress is in freefall. 'This damage to the nation's health', Marmot writes, 'need not have happened.' What seismic event triggered a sharp decline in the health and longevity of those lower down the social ladder?

The team analysed potential explanations for the reduction in life expectancy. Maybe we've reached peak length of life? No. Perhaps there was a bad flu season that increased the mortality statistics? Again, no. The simple answer offered is austerity, an economic policy that aims to reduce government budget deficits by reducing public spending. Austerity affects the poor more severely than the better off. During the period of the report there was a 40 per cent reduction in welfare spending for families, pushing more children into poverty and worsening their long-term health and economic prospects. This is the exact opposite of what we should have done, as shown by the Heckman Equation.

The Heckman Equation

Professor James Heckman is a Nobel Prize-winning economist who has shown that 'the highest rate of economic returns comes from the earliest investments in children'. The most efficient and effective place for a government to allocate its resources is in pregnancy and early life. Policies that invest in children's education and wellbeing are the best way to support the future stability and resilience of the country.

And, of course, early childhood learning *depends on early child brain development.* Investing in the health and nutrition of pregnant women and their children is the most economically rational and effective strategy for any sensible, serious government. But it is important to acknowledge that the widening health disparities harm the entire country, not just the poor. For example, a recent report conducted by PwC for Impact on Urban Health showed that expanding free school meal provision would result in substantial benefits to the economy over 20 years, including increased cost savings to schools, increased lifetime earnings and contributions, and savings to the NHS.

Projected Outcomes of Expanding FSM to Families

Scenario	Cost of implementation (£bn)	Core benefits (£bn)	Wider benefits (£bn)	Total combined benefit (£bn)
Expanding FSM to all families in receipt of Universal Credit	6.4	8.9	16.2	25.1
Universal FSM to all pupils in state-funded schools	24.2	41.3	58.2	99.5

Human capital

These broader economic benefits are a function of 'human capital', the quasi-dystopian process of estimating someone's lifetime economic value. The government offers the following definition: 'the stock of skills, knowledge and experience of an individual or population, which can productively be applied in the economy'. As such, human capital is considered 'one of the main drivers of economic growth'.

Nutrition quality, then, is a lever of human capital. Nutrition quality determines someone's physical and mental health. Their health status determines their productivity. Their productivity determines their economic value. To this end government intervention that improves the food environment and the nutritional status of the nation needn't be thought of as overly restrictive and intrusive regulations. Rather, they are shrewd and judicious long-term economic policies. Health is a human capital asset.

Moreover, mental health is a significant determinant of adult economic productivity, not just in terms of the impact of time off work for mental health reasons, but because mental ill health can affect important productivity factors like concentration, motivation and stress tolerance. Most mental health conditions emerge during adolescence, influenced by the status of current and early life nutrition on brain structure, mood and stress resilience (as well as non-nutrition factors).

The American Special Supplemental Nutrition Program for Women, Infants, and Children (WIC) is a federal programme that provides state funding for 'supplemental foods, health care referrals and nutrition education for low-income pregnant, breastfeeding and non-breastfeeding postpartum women, and to infants and children up to age 5 who are found to be at nutritional risk'. In a 2018 review of the outcomes of the programme, researchers found that participation was associated with a 5 per cent reduced risk of being diagnosed with ADHD, a 5.1 per cent lower chance of being diagnosed with other common mental health conditions, and a 7.9 per cent lowered probability of having to repeat a school year.

Healthier children become healthier, more productive adults. The World Bank reports that early nutrition programmes increase school completion and raise adult wages by between 5 and 50 per cent, helping to lift people out of poverty. This is why children going hungry, and the cognitive and psychological harm that comes with that, is not just a moral failing but socioeconomic recklessness.

Hidden hunger

In January 2021, the Scottish Conservative Party suspended one of their candidates for comments he made about those who used food banks. Following a Channel 4 programme on food poverty, Craig Ross took to his podcast to explain that those using food banks were 'far from starving' and that 'if anything, their biggest risk is not starvation, it's diabetes'. These kinds of disparaging comments are not unusual and pop up on social media whenever food bank usage is mentioned. I get the sense that these complainers are rather disappointed; the poor people aren't doing the job of being poor quite well enough. What they want, it seems, is a barefoot, emaciated, Dickensian urchin in rags, with hands outstretched in supplication. That's the vision of poverty we've all grown up with, that's how you know for sure that someone is (deserving) poor.

What comments like this betray, other than a fundamental lack of compassion, is ignorance of the phenomenon of hidden hunger, which is the existence of micronutrient deficiencies in the presence of macro-nutrient availability or abundance. That is to say, someone is getting enough energy (calories) but not enough vitamins, minerals, fibre or essential fats. Their body has sufficient energy stores but their brains are starving.

FOOD BANKS

In the reporting period 2011–12, 128,697 people received emergency food parcels from the Trussell Trust network of food banks. In 2021–22 the number of recipients was 2,173,158.

The added nutritional burden for those using food banks is that the majority of foods donated are, by definition, ultra-processed, in order to be shelf-stable. Since people living in food-insecure homes are already the most undernourished, they are then at risk of further malnourishment.

Additionally, as the poverty crisis continues to eat into household disposable income and savings, fewer people are able to afford to donate to food banks. Many will be destitute without government action.

The cycle of poverty

Food, brain development, mental health and poverty are inextricably linked. Income inequality translates to health inequality: the lower your socioeconomic status, the worse your diet, the poorer your health, the poorer your children's health. We have seen in the early chapters how important a nutritious diet is for the baby's brain development. These advantages compound and accumulate over time. What might be a few points on a classroom test at the age of seven could be the difference between the child being put forward for a higher-performing secondary school or being considered for a valuable internship or jobs programme. Furthermore, future income is linked to IQ, which is tied to brain development. More than this, happiness is linked to IQ and this relationship is mediated by factors like wealth and health.

But don't just take my word for it. In a review paper published in 2020, scientists wrote:

> *The cycle of poverty and malnutrition appears to be intergenerational. Evidence suggests that malnourished women are at a higher risk of having malnourished children and this creates an intergenerational effect. It is imperative to intervene early in life in order to maximize the effectiveness of interventions and break the cycle . . . In other words, the interventions need to reach the poorest of the poor to break the cycle of malnutrition and poverty.*

While these researchers were taking a view of global poverty, we know that these dynamics are present and persistent in the UK. Malnutrition compromises an individual's cognitive capacity and potential. Consequently, their productivity is impaired and, therefore, their earning potential. With a lower income they (in our current food environment) are less able to afford nutritious food, further depriving their brain (and body) and increasing their vulnerability to psychiatric illness and neurodegeneration. Poor nutrition is both a cause and consequence of poverty. Good health is increasingly a trapping of wealth.

There is no economic justification for not extending the eligibility for free school meals. Nor is there any sensible moral opposition. Correspondingly, the disinvestment in programmes and support for poorer children and their families is an abandonment of a huge proportion of the population by the state.

The nutritional and health inequalities faced by children from poor households put them at a neurological disadvantage *from the moment of conception*. From 'before the beginning' they are set on a trajectory of unfulfilled potential. For any government to then turn

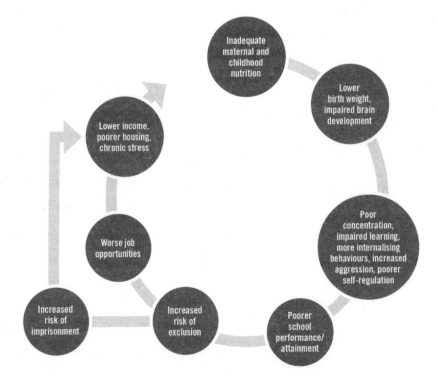

around, when that child is 20, 25, 30 years of age, and say 'you are here entirely through your own choice' is repugnant. If we (society and the government) are not deliberate in systematically dismantling the notion that the poor 'choose' to be so, or that the wealthy are better-quality cornflakes who are 'born to lead', in reigniting the mechanisms of social mobility and reducing health and educational inequality, we are poised to cement those who simply have the misfortune of being born to poor families as members of a permanent underclass. Though, as you will read in the next chapter, we might already be there.

CHAPTER 11

CRIME AND NOURISHMENT – THE PRISON NUTRITION STUDIES

WITH WEARYING PREDICTABILITY, every new British election cycle or leadership contest generates reheated promises to get 'tough on crime'. The thing is . . . the UK is already pretty darn tough on crime. The average length of a custodial sentence has been steadily increasing since 2009, when it was 13.7 months. By 2019 that figure was 18.9 months. Nonetheless, the Conservative Party's winning 2019 manifesto included a promise to introduce 'tougher sentencing for criminals'. This included extending the minimum portion of their sentence spent behind bars from half to two-thirds.

Having worked in the prison estate I would be more sympathetic to this strategy if there was any evidence that it actually worked to make people safer and reduce crime. But simply, there isn't. Instead, according to a recent systematic review, we have the highest reoffending rates *in the world*. Whatever these longer sentences are doing, they're not deterring people from committing crimes. In fact, longer sentences increase the rate of recidivism, and it's not difficult to understand why. The longer you are in prison, the longer you are out of work, the more likely you are to lose your housing, and the more time you have to build relationships with other criminals.

What longer sentences are effective at doing, though, is increasing the prison population. As of August 2022 the UK had a prison population of 81,207, with a further 2,121 individuals sentenced in the community under home curfew. This gives us the third highest prison population in Europe, only behind such authoritarian regimes as Russia and Turkey. And the Ministry of Justice recently predicted that the prison population would grow by nearly 25 per cent by 2026. We truly do strive to be 'world-beating'.

These high and growing levels of incarceration mean that our prisons are increasingly crowded. HM Chief Inspector of Prisons for England and Wales described overcrowding as a 'significant' problem in around 60 per cent of the prisons inspected in 2015–16. And crowded prisons are also dangerous prisons. While the number of suicides was down in the 12 months to June 2022 (a prisoner died from self-inflicted injuries every five and a half days compared to every four and a half days in the previous 12 months), self-harm increased. Figures for 2022 showed that incidents of self-harm in women's prisons doubled in the preceding year. In general, women self-harm at seven times the rate of men in prison. Assaults on staff went up 8 per cent in the 12 months to March 2022, with 7,599 recorded incidents, while serious prisoner-on-prisoner assaults increased by 14 per cent. Perhaps unsurprisingly, the use of force against prisoners has doubled in the last decade. UK prisons are increasingly violent and dangerous places to live and work.

This worrying situation was largely exacerbated by cuts to funding that began in 2010, with prison spending hitting its lowest (in real terms) around 2016. Staff numbers were cut by 30 per cent during this period. I was working in a prison at the time and I watched in dismay as experienced (and therefore more expensive) prison officers left in their droves, to be replaced with young and inexperienced newbies. I would speak with officers on the wings who were desperate and exhausted, and at times understandably resentful that I was there offering psychological support to prisoners. Where was their support? Despite recent increased investment, funding is still currently 14 per cent below 2009–10 levels. In spite of this the government is going ahead with plans to create 20,000 additional prison places within the next few years, which, again, will do nothing to reduce crime rates. It's not entirely clear where the money will come from to house all of these prisoners, at an average cost of £48,162. That figure, by the way, the highest cost per prisoner in Europe, has been rising year on year since 2015, partly because prisoners now present with more complex needs. The prison population is aging (hello longer sentences and high reoffending rates), which brings increased physical health needs, as well as the ever-present drug, alcohol and mental health issues.

Mental Illness in Prison

The Bethlem Royal Hospital, from where the derogatory term 'bedlam' is derived, was established in London in 1247. Initially built as a priory, by around 1460 it was an asylum for the 'insane'. Aside from Bethlem there were few provisions for the care of the mentally ill during this period, leading to huge growth in the 'trade in lunacy', a plethora of unregulated, private, profit-making establishments where the unwell were held and the public could pay to observe them as 'entertainment'.

Though (mainstream) psychiatric care has moved on enormously since the early days of 'bedlam', something of their essence lives on, I fear. In my opinion, it would be neither unfair nor inaccurate to think of prisons as enormous old-style psychiatric wards both in terms of the rates of mental illness and the lack of government oversight.

'Government does not know how many people in prison have a mental illness, how much it is spending on mental health in prisons or whether it is achieving its objectives. It is therefore hard to see how Government can be achieving value for money in its efforts to improve the mental health and wellbeing of prisoners.' Those are the opening lines of a 2017 report from the National Audit Office, an independent parliamentary body that oversees and audits government departments. It continues: 'Her Majesty's Prisons and Probation Service (HMPPS), NHS England and Public Health England have set ambitious objectives for providing mental health services but do not collect enough or good enough data to understand whether they are meeting them.'

Other sources, such as independent research teams, do collect prison mental health data and they find that there is a dramatic overrepresentation of mental illness in prisons compared to illness rates in the general population. A 2017 article in the *Lancet Psychiatry* estimates that 'two-thirds [66 per cent] of prisoners suffer from personality disorders, roughly half suffer from depression and anxiety, and one in twelve suffer from psychosis'. This compares to 4.4 per cent, 7.8 per cent and one in 100, respectively, in the general population (though drug use in prison may account for some of the increased psychosis). People in prison are 33 per cent more likely to have had adverse childhood experiences (see page 137) than the general population. In fact, despite making up less than 1 per cent of the general population, people who were in care as children make up nearly 25 per cent of the prison population.

Ineffective. Dangerous. Expensive. And Only Getting Worse

But here we are, year after year, with the same uninformed, harmful, predictable policy promises. It is an appalling state of affairs brought about because none of our politicians have the courage to look at the reality of the causes of crime.

So, what *would* reduce offending rates? Let's look at the risk factors.

Though accurate prevalence rates are difficult to ascertain due to the nature of the crime and the victims, a recent survey by children's charity the NSPCC reported that 7 per cent of girls and 2.6 per cent of boys had experienced contact childhood sexual abuse by the age of 17. A systematic review of 24 countries' prevalence data similarly found rates of 8–31 per cent for girls and 3–17 per cent for boys. In contrast, an American study of inmates at county jails found that 59 per cent of male prisoners had experienced childhood sexual abuse. Other work has put that figure at a conservative 40 per cent. Around 30 per cent of female offenders report being victims of sexual abuse in childhood, and 66 per cent of the women who self-harm in prison report being victims of childhood sexual abuse.

The educational experiences of prisoners also differ significantly from the general population. According to the National Literacy Trust between 12 and 16.4 per cent of adults in England and Wales have poor literacy skills. Up to 90 per cent of young offenders have below average language ability, and 62 per cent have a reading age of five. Such poor reading ability makes it incredibly difficult to engage with rehabilitation and educational programmes. Some 42 per cent of prisoners had been permanently excluded or expelled from school; 24 per cent had been in care.

One of the leading risk factors for later incarceration is having a parent imprisoned. So, as well as not deterring crime, longer, tougher sentences actually increase intergenerational criminal behaviour. You couldn't make it up.

Typically, there is a high prevalence of childhood trauma and psychiatric illness in incarcerated populations. And long, excessively punitive sentences simply perpetuate that intergenerational cycle. Even if you don't care about the plight of prisoners, you perhaps care about the billions of taxpayers' money being spent on a system that, objectively, is not fit for purpose. All of the emerging evidence suggests that, rather than futile and counter-productive pledges to get 'tough on crime', the most effective way to reduce offending would be to protect at-risk children.

And so you'd think – with all the self-harm, the assaults on hardworking staff, the mental illness, the sheer expense – that the government would be interested in anything that could help. You might then think it inconceivable that the Home Office might already know of an intervention that costs mere pennies a day per prisoner that could reduce violence in prisons by 30 per cent. You would perhaps think it impossible that they have had that information for over 20 years, and done precisely nothing with it. Imagine having a treatment that could reliably eliminate an illness by 30 per cent and ignoring it. What would you even call that? Negligent? Callous? Incompetent? Well, do I have a story for you.

Prison Studies

What I call 'the prison studies' are a group of international nutrition trials (outlined on the next page) that report remarkably similar outcomes of the effects of improved nutrition on violence in prisons. In each of these studies nutritional supplements were provided and compared to a placebo. In each of these studies violent incidents were reduced by about 30 per cent in the supplement group compared to the placebo group. Now, we've seen this figure before: this is the same magnitude of effect in the reduction of playground fights in the schools that provided hungry children with breakfast. In prison, at current levels, that could translate to over 2,500 *fewer* assaults on staff, as well as savings in relation to employee sick leave, improved staff retention and reduced compensation pay-outs.

Author	Year	Method	Participants	Outcome
Schoenthaler et al.	1997	Randomised Placebo-controlled Double-blind Multivitamin and mineral supplement 12 weeks	62 US young male offenders	28% fewer violent infractions in the supplemented group
Gesch et al.	2002	Randomised Placebo-controlled Double-blind Multivitamin and mineral supplement 2-week minimum	231 UK adult male prisoners	35% reduction in violence in the supplemented group
Zaalberg et al.	2010	Randomised Placebo-controlled Triple-blind Multivitamins, minerals and omega-3 4–12 weeks	221 Dutch adult male prisoners	34% reduction in violence in the supplemented group, 14% increase in violence in the placebo group
Raine et al.	2020	Randomised Placebo-controlled Double-blind Omega-3, vitamin D and antioxidants 12 weeks	145 Singaporean young offenders	Reduced self-reported antisocial behaviour and reactive impulsive aggression

I spoke to Dr Bernard Gesch, the lead researcher on the 2002 UK prison study. He said:

This is a very easy way to prevent offending. You must have come across the Dutch Hunger Studies [see box below] where they are now on the second cohort and they are still seeing effects on behaviour. Now, if you're looking at lab animals, if you introduce a nutritional insult, you can see changes over three generations; it takes three generations of improved nutrition to breed that out. So this is potentially highly cost-effective because if you improve the nutrition now, you could be benefiting in three generations.

THE DUTCH HUNGER WINTER

During the final winter of the Second World War, Germany blockaded the Netherlands, cutting off supplies of food and fuel. The resulting famine caused the death of at least 18,000 people.

Between November 1943 and February 1947, 2,414 children were born in the now defunct Wilhelmina Gasthuis hospital to mothers who had been pregnant during the famine, and some shortly before or after the famine conditions. This group of children comprise the Dutch Famine Birth Cohort, providing an opportunity to examine the impact of famine on pregnancy and later health. They were followed up first in 1994 and several more times in the intervening years. This very special study/group has given researchers a rare opportunity to trace the impact of in utero stress and undernutrition on the health not just of the children, but also their descendants. The findings to date have been fascinating. Exposure to famine in utero has permanent effects on health. For example, these individuals have a higher risk of heart disease compared to matched controls. They also have poorer glucose control, and the women are more likely to carry fat around the waist. The bodies of those exposed to famine in the womb hold on to fat more readily. It seems that the low availability of energy during pregnancy primed these children's DNA for the same after birth. It's as if the body said, 'Okay, there isn't much food around so we need to do everything we can to hold on to fat and sugar.' The nutritional exposure in the womb programmed their DNA. This 'thrifty gene expression' is an adaptation to increase their chances of surviving in an environment with limited food availability.

However, in this case, the conditions in the womb did not persist after birth; the war ended, the country was liberated and food became more available. In this environmental context the genetic programming that would have helped them to survive in famine conditions became a hindrance, increasing their risk of heart disease. And the impacts persist down the generations. Children born to the men who were famine babies have a higher BMI. The children born to the famine cohort women developed more fat as babies. This and other studies remind us that the quality of a woman's nutrition during pregnancy affects not only her and her child, but her grandchildren and perhaps even her great-grandchildren.

Violence is a scourge on our society. Whether it's the playground bully who can strip children of their self-esteem, domestic abuse or other assaults that change or end lives. We often think about violence as being a feature of someone's personality. A character flaw. So it is utterly remarkable that something as unremarkable as a nutritional supplement could have such profound effects.

That said, by now we should not be too surprised that nutritional status should have an effect on behavioural outcomes. First, the brain and its neurotransmitters are *made of nutrients*. We also know that the brain has a high nutrient and energy demand. And we have seen both that nutrient deficiencies impair brain structure and that supplements and improved diet can enhance cognition in children and adults.

Relevant to the prison population, there is also abundant evidence of an association between poor micronutrient status and mental illness. A systematic review of 28 studies found a significant inverse correlation between levels of folate and vitamin D and first-episode psychosis (the first time someone experiences a psychotic episode).

Interestingly, in the Raine et al. study, improvements were also seen in the parents' behaviour. The researchers had not accounted for this unexpected result so they are unsure what caused it. It is possible that the parents were drinking the supplement drinks intended for the children. But, plausibly, calmer children simply result in calmer parents and fewer points of emotional escalation.

Another trial is currently underway to explore the role of omega-3 and prisoner aggression in Australia on the basis of these studies and prior evidence showing a relationship between lower omega-3 status and greater tendency to aggression in Australian prisoners.

Ideally, nutritional improvement would come in the form of food. However, the benefit of supplements over wholefoods in these studies is that it allows for 'blinding' – participants do not know whether they are getting the real supplement or the placebo. It's virtually impossible to blind people to actual food; you know whether you are eating an apple or a sausage roll. In each study, at the end of the trial period violence in those taking the supplements was significantly reduced. What is important about these studies is that they were all randomised, blinded and placebo-controlled. This methodology, which aims to reduce the potential for bias in clinical research, is considered the best way to test the efficacy of a treatment. Indeed, it is the 'gold standard' means of discerning whether a drug or other treatment really does what it says on the tin. Finally, there were no reported side effects of taking the supplements – in other words, it was a safe intervention. What this indicates is that improved nutrition presents a cheap, low-risk and accessible opportunity to reduce the growing rates of violence in UK prisons. In an era in which we are seeing record levels of self-injury and suicide, this could equate to lives saved as well as safer prisons for staff.

Independent of violence, improving nutrition in prisons could provide other benefits. Up to 90 per cent of prisoners are thought to have a diagnosable mental health condition. In this area, there is a growing scientific consensus on the importance of good nutrition for mental wellbeing. You will read in the next chapter how nutrition also affects conditions like depression and PTSD (post-traumatic stress disorder). Again, it is unlikely that better food will resolve all of these issues, but it may meaningfully reduce the levels of distress and the burden on prison security and healthcare staff.

I wondered whether the cost of supplementation was the reason change was not implemented. Not so. An economic analysis commissioned by the Home Office following the results of the Gesch et al. study showed that providing prisoners with supplements would cost around £40 per prisoner per year. And while providing more fresh (perishable) produce may cost more than the current highly processed fare, similar to what we saw with the downstream benefits of free school meals, those costs are likely to be offset by savings on security and staff turnover. For a potential 30 per cent reduction in violence, improved physical and mental health, fewer riots and better staff retention, improved nutrition would seem like a worthwhile investment. But Dr Gesch has struggled for years to have the UK government act on his (and others') research.

> *I don't feel I've hung my boots up just yet, but when you keep bashing your head against a brick wall eventually you get tired and a headache.*

As a nutrition researcher with decades of experience, I asked Dr Gesch about his fears for the future.

> *KW: What are you afraid might be down the line for us if we don't sort this out now?*

> *BG: If you look at mental illness, for example, it has overtaken heart disease as the single biggest cost across Europe. It was predicted that children's mental health problems would double from 1980 and I think we're well ahead of that curve already.*

Prison: The Nutritional Wild West

There are surprisingly few regulations on the quality of prison food in the UK. The Prison Rules stipulate simply that prison food should be 'wholesome, nutritious, well prepared and served, reasonably varied and sufficient in quantity'. In reality this stipulation is broad to the point of meaningless and subject to wide interpretation since terms like 'wholesome' and 'nutritious' have no clinical definition. For simply supplying the macronutrients carbohydrates, protein and fat, it could technically be claimed that a peanut and caramel chocolate bar constituted 'nutritious'. Additionally, prison food in the UK is provided by private contractors, meaning that profit margins and shareholder returns factor into the variety and quality of food provided. The national catering contract for UK prisons is currently held by Bidfood UK. In 2020 the company's pre-tax profits nearly doubled from £28.9 million to £55.1 million. They were later able to secure another lucrative government contract to supply food packs to people forced to shield during the pandemic. Bidfood's parent company BFS Group paid out £30.5 million in dividends to shareholders while at the same time taking advantage of the government's furlough scheme. Clearly, they were doing something right, fiscally, if not morally. But there's no such thing as a free lunch; those shareholder profits have to come from somewhere. Indeed, typically, the meals on offer are highly refined, ultra-processed food of low-nutrient density. The standard breakfast pack is composed of a 30g (variety pack size) box of breakfast cereal, sachets of coffee, tea and sugar, and a carton of milk, white and sometimes brown bread for toast, jam and margarine. Lunch is usually a white bread sandwich, biscuits and a piece of fruit. The images posted online by serving male prisoners depict the reality of the ultra-processed dinners provided. A sausage roll served with plain white pasta, a pasty and potatoes, rather dry-looking battered fish and chips. These meals do not provide adequate fibre or nutrients for optimal brain and mental health. Neither prisoners, prison staff, nor the public benefit from cheap prison food. And yet.

According to nutrition charity the Food Foundation it costs £5.99

per day for an adult to meet the UK's Eatwell healthy diet recommendations. An average of just £2 is spent on prisoners' meals. Even accounting for economies of scale, it seems unlikely that £2 is sufficient to provide three filling and nutritionally adequate meals for an adult.

Finally, aside from the colossal waste of human potential and money, this research should unsettle you because it shakes the foundations of a cornerstone of our judicial system: free will. We have a justice system that is predicated on volition; the assumption that we have conscious control over our behaviours, such that if we engage in violent or criminal acts we have done so of our own *choice*. We made a wrong decision and therefore are deserving of the consequences. The fly in the ointment of volition is that it assumes that the machinery of decision-making – the brain – is working properly. What these well-conducted studies seriously call into question is how well an undernourished brain can work. If someone is less prone to violence when they have an adequate intake of nutrients, how culpable are they for their previous violent behaviour? Especially if they had no idea that what they were (or were not) eating was affecting their brain in this way?

GOVERNMENT NEGLIGENCE?

Earlier I asked you whether the government's failure to follow up and act on the original prison study's data could be considered negligent.

Legally, for someone to bring a case of negligence under English law they have to demonstrate that:

1. An entity owed them a duty of care
2. The entity breached that duty of care
3. They suffered a loss due to that breach of duty of care

The Prison Service certainly owes a duty of care to prisoners and staff to take all reasonable measures to ensure the environment is a safe place to live and work. It seems to me that in a situation where a member of staff was injured by a prisoner, a case could be made that the combination of understaffing and the failure to introduce easy-to-implement nutritional interventions that could significantly reduce the risk of violence could constitute a breach.

Is it reasonable for the Prison Service to supplement prisoners? Well, considering that the Prison Service control the majority of prisoners' nutrition and prisoners are a nutritionally at-risk group, I think the answer is yes.

Would supplementation be a 'reasonable' expense? My crude cost-benefit analysis indicates that for a few pennies a day prisoners' mental and physical health would improve and violence would reduce. Neither staff (nor prisoners) could be expected to know that violence could be reduced so easily but, crucially, this is information that is available to the government, so it might be fairly easily argued that they showed a lack of adequate precautions to ensure safety. Proving that the breach directly caused the injury would be difficult but it would certainly be an interesting test case.

The failure of the government to act on the outcomes of the prison studies is astonishing. To me it speaks of an utter contempt not just for prisoners, but for the people who work in prisons and their families. Why would you not implement such a cheap, easy and effective strategy? Is it simply a lack of interest? Who benefits from having more offenders held in increasingly dangerous prisons . . . other than those who have secured lucrative prison procurement and building contracts?

TAKE ACTION

Help raise awareness of the prison studies and the dramatic reduction in violence they reveal by either telling two people you know or downloading a template for you to post on your preferred social media account by going to https://www.kimberley wilson.co/crime-and-nourishment.

CHAPTER 12

NUTRITION AND MOOD

LET'S TURN NOW to one of the most prevalent and pressing mental health conditions. Depression is one of the leading causes of disease burden in the world and you will have read in the opening section of the book about the high rates of treatment-resistant depression. With the failure of the serotonin hypothesis, researchers and mental health practitioners across the world are left looking for other effective treatments for this debilitating condition.

Epidemiological data provides clear evidence for the relationship between diet and depression: the lower the proportion of UPFDs in your diet, the lower the risk and severity of depression. However, while observations can tell us about the strength of an association, it can't tell us for sure that one thing leads to another. Fortunately, a crop of new experimental studies is providing the evidence for a causal relationship between poor diet and depression.

The most famous of these is the SMILES (Supporting the Modification of lifestyle in Lowered Emotional States) trial, which took 67 people with a diagnosis of depression and a poor diet. Participants were randomly assigned to either a nutritional intervention group, where they were supported to enjoy a Mediterranean-style diet (fewer ultra-processed foods, more fruit, veg and fibre), or a befriending control group (befriending is known to improve depression). After 12 weeks of nutritional improvement those in the nutritional intervention group

185

were four times more likely to be in remission than those in the befriending group. They also had reduced severity of anxiety symptoms.

Though women have a greater overall risk of depression compared to men, men are less likely to ask for or be referred to psychological therapy, reducing their treatment opportunities. Young men are also substantially more likely to die by suicide, for which depression is a major risk factor. So, developing additional treatment options that are acceptable and accessible to young men is crucial. Could diet help? A 12-week Australian study published in 2022 suggests it could. In the trial, 72 men aged 18–25, with moderate to severe depression, were randomly assigned to receive either three online sessions of clinical nutritionist-led dietary improvement (based on the dietary recommendations for Spain) or befriending. Befriending in this study involved talking about things they enjoyed and leisure activities. In the nutrition group the men were supported to reduce their consumption of fast foods, sugar and red meat (just three servings a week of these foods), and increase their intake of brightly coloured vegetables, legumes/beans, wholegrains, oily fish, olive oil and raw unsalted nuts. The men were assessed on their adherence to a Mediterranean diet and completed validated scales of depression and quality of life, at baseline, six weeks and 12 weeks. At the end of the three months, the men in the diet group improved significantly more than the befriending group. In fact, at the end of the study, 36 per cent of the men in the diet group had depression scores that were 'low or minimal'. They also reported improved sleep, concentration and energy. The researchers report that the men were keen to continue with the dietary improvement after the end of the study, indicating that this is a feasible intervention for young men who can otherwise find it difficult to open up about their mental health difficulties.

In another study with a similar design 152 people with self-reported depression received either food hampers for three months and fish oil supplements for six months, or attended befriending. At three months the diet group saw a greater reduction in depression and improved quality of life, and these benefits were sustained at six months. Impressively, the reduction in depression was proportional to the level of adherence to a healthy diet, mirroring the observational data.

In these studies, data on the mechanisms of action were not collected but previous research suggests that improved nutrition could reduce nutritional deficiencies, improve neurotransmitter synthesis and provide substrate for the gut microbiome (see chapter 8), all of which can support brain function. Together, the observational and trial data tell a story of how poor diets are contributing to the burden of depression. Nutritionally poor UPFs make up over half the diet of UK adults and up to 80 per cent for children. Elsewhere these links between diet and depression have led to changes in official health recommendations.

In 2020 the Royal Australian and New Zealand College of Psychiatrists updated their practice guidelines (similar to the UK's NICE guidelines) for mood disorders to include nutrition improvement as 'essential' to the management of depression. This means that patients in the Antipodes who present to their GP with the symptoms of depression should be offered information on the potential role of their diets on their depression symptoms and how to improve their nutrition to support their recovery.

This evidence leads us to reassess our understanding of the underlying causes of depression. We have seen how the serotonin hypothesis was insufficient. So where does that leave us? I believe the 'inflammation hypothesis' is a much better explanatory model for depression. The inflammation hypothesis proposes that elevated or dysfunctional immune activity (inflammation) drives many of the symptoms of depression. For example, inflammation can:

- Loosen the tight junctions of the BBB (see page 200).
- Inhibit brain cell growth and function.
- Reduce the availability of serotonin and dopamine.
- Increase the production of neurotoxic compounds.
- Increase oxidative stress.
- Impair memory and concentration.
- Impair sleep.

While psychological, chemical and viral stress can induce these effects, so can a poor diet. A tool called the dietary inflammatory index (DII) assesses the potential of a diet to promote inflammation and has been used in numerous clinical trials. The emerging consensus is that the higher the inflammatory potential of a person's diet, the worse their brain function will tend to be. A large prospective study that followed over 26,000 people for an average of five years found that those with a more pro-inflammatory diet had a greater risk of developing depression.

According to the DII, the foods and nutrients with the most anti-inflammatory potential are: fibre, beta-carotene (found in brightly coloured vegetables), garlic, ginger, iron, turmeric, vitamins A, C, D and E (fruit, vegetables, oily fish, nuts), green and black tea, flavones and flavanols (berries), and omega-3 fats (oily fish and seafood). Over-all diets that score low on these foods and that are high in saturated, trans- and omega-6 fats and low in omega-3 fats are linked to higher levels of inflammatory markers. Correspondingly, there is a direct association between the inflammatory potential of a person's diet and their risk of depression.

Given this clear and robust association any public health intervention that is designed to reduce the burden of depression *must* include policies that effectively improve public nutrition. Treatment interventions that ignore diet quality are just mopping the floor without turning off the tap.

Stress

While we are adapted to manage (and sometimes grow from) small doses of manageable stress, chronic or overwhelming stress erodes wellbeing and sets the stage for depression and related conditions. Three-quarters of Brits report experiencing overwhelming stress, so the news that nutritional interventions can help is welcome and relevant. Research from Professor Julia Rucklidge's team in New Zealand shows how valuable it can be. Building on previous results showing that taking a broad-spectrum nutritional supplement (one that contains a wide range of vitamins and minerals) reduces stress and anxiety (and even leads to remission) in people with ADHD, this research group wanted to see whether supplements would also benefit the general population.

Following the powerful earthquakes in Christchurch in 2011 participants were split into three groups and took either medium or high doses of a supplement called CNE for four weeks or Berocca. This widely available commercial supplement was used as a comparison because its efficacy was established in previous trials. A group of people who had applied for the trial and then decided not to take part (so were not taking supplements) provided a control group. All participants completed scales of stress, anxiety, depression, trauma, overall functioning and provided food diaries. At the end of four weeks the research team found that all three treatment groups improved in stress, mood, anxiety and energy. That is to say that additional nutritional support following the stressful event was helpful for everyone, but other differences between the groups emerged. The high-dose CNE group had fewer intrusive thoughts (distressing, involuntary thoughts that seem to just pop into the mind and can be difficult to shake off), and reported better mood and less anxiety compared to the Berocca group. At baseline, 70 of the 116 participants (60 per cent) had probable PTSD. At four weeks, only 19 per cent of the participants in the treatment groups had probable PTSD, compared with 48 per cent of the unsupplemented controls. At follow-up a month later, those who stayed on the supplements showed greater continued improvement in depression, anxiety, stress and energy compared with those who came off them. These results point to some important features of micronutrients:

1. They are effective.
2. They are accessible and easy to administer.
3. They are cheap.
4. They have a low risk of side effects.

Those at risk of PTSD, anxiety or burnout might benefit from ensuring adequate intake of a broad spectrum of micronutrients, whether through supplementation or, ideally, a nutrient-dense wholefood diet.

NUTRIENTS ALONGSIDE MEDICATION

As I mentioned earlier, despite high prescription rates, antidepressants aren't as effective as we need them to be. The growing body of evidence for the role of food and nutrients in supporting mental health raises the question of whether nutrients could improve drug efficacy. A systematic review and meta-analysis published in 2016 says yes. After reviewing 40 studies they identified a moderate to strong beneficial effect of omega-3 (particularly EPA), as well as positive results for methylfolate (folic acid) and vitamin D alongside medication. There were also no major adverse effects of supplementation recorded. This is great, potentially life-enhancing news for patients.

Cortisol

It is much more common to talk about cortisol as a stress hormone because it is a major coordinator of the fight/flight/freeze response. However, one of cortisol's key roles is the regulation of blood sugar, and for this reason I think it more than deserves its place in a conversation about food and mood. As blood glucose drops cortisol increases, promoting the release of glucose from the body's stores. This helps to ensure the brain-body has sufficient energy to face the perceived challenge, but it has a downside. States of stress bias our brains to think negatively and emotionally, rather than in a rational and optimistic manner, and this can have adverse effects on mood and decision-making.

In an unusual study design, researchers enlisted 107 long-married (average 12 years) couples to provide morning and evening glucose measurements for three weeks. To measure aggression the participants were asked to insert pins into a voodoo doll of their spouse, depending on how angry they were with them. The team found a correlation between cortisol levels and the number of pins inserted. In a separate experiment, individuals with higher cortisol also blasted their partner with louder noises, and for longer periods.

Valence

Though we tend to think of our decisions as higher-order brain functions that are largely rational and objective, this view is not supported by the research evidence. Our body provides our brain with constant feedback on its state – energy levels, pain, hydration, metabolites, inflammation, etc. The brain receives a message from the body that sounds something like 'all is well' or 'I'm not happy'. This signal of pleasantness or unpleasantness is called valence, and the brain combines this with information about energy levels to come up with what psychologists call our 'affective states' (see diagram below).

So, your emotional states aren't simply a response to your thoughts or our psychological interactions with the outside world. They are a synthesis of these factors PLUS information about the *state of your body*. It is very difficult for your brain to generate an instance of good

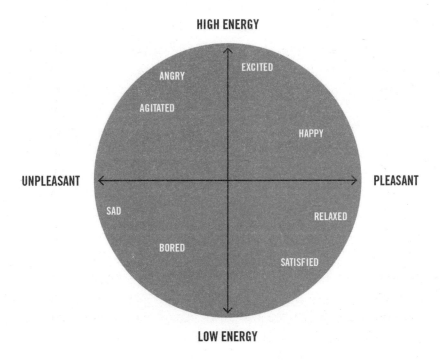

mood if your body is sending loud signals that things are not right. Therefore, if your body is straining under the pressure of burdens like nutritional deficiencies, diet-induced inflammation and high blood glucose, your mood *will be affected*. Conversely, a well-nourished body will be more resilient to stress and low mood, conveying positive valence signals to your brain.

A TALE OF TWO BRAINS

Though she experienced many of the struggles of young adulthood – break-ups with partners and friends, exam and work stress, the death of a colleague – Anya seemed largely resilient. She would feel sad and occasionally overwhelmed, but it never got to the stage where she felt she was at 'breaking point'. In fact, she became known in her office as someone who was able to work well under pressure, which contributed to her being selected for promotion. This sits with the evidence that people who habitually consume a minimally pro-cessed wholefood diet have a reduced risk of developing depression and increased stress resilience.

Sadly, the bouts of low mood that had started in Mia's twenties continued into her thirties. She saw a couple of therapists for a while and, though she found it helpful for making sense of some of her relationships, it didn't really seem to shift the 'unsettled' feeling that she always had. She just always felt that 'something was wrong', even though events in her life were, objectively, going well. Eventu-ally, her GP diagnosed her with depression and anxiety and started her on a course of antidepressants. She wasn't sure whether they helped but the idea that there was an 'imbalance in her brain' was the only thing that made sense to her. Initially she planned to take them for only six months, but she stayed on them for several years (around 40 per cent of patients prescribed antidepressants remain on them long term). Things would always be a bit worse when she was stressed, like when she had big work deadlines. At these times she would also find herself craving sweet foods like chocolate biscuits and sweet coffee drinks. Sometimes she drank so much coffee that it started to interfere with her sleep. So she would 'need' more coffee the next day . . . When she noticed that all the biscuits were making it difficult to manage her weight, she would try dieting. The thing that seemed most effective for her was cutting carbs. Mia didn't like many vegetables so during these periods she would eat a lot of meat, cheese and eggs and the occasional salad. She would lose weight but found this way of eating hard to sustain for more than a few weeks at a time. In the end she decided it would be better for her physical and mental wellbeing to shift to a less demanding role. This move relieved some of the external pressure but didn't really help with the 'unsettled' feeling. She felt disappointed that she just 'couldn't keep up'. It reminded her of how she had felt back at school and the teacher who'd told her she could do better if she just 'applied herself'.

Mia's experience is, sadly, the more familiar one. One that, I hope you can see, has its roots in the outmoded view of the mind as separate from the body. The unsettled feeling is negative valence, her body telling her something is not right, which is interpreted as psychological distress. It's likely that addressing some of her body-brain's nutritional needs would have provided some relief, even adjunct to her prescribed medication. It would certainly have been worth a try. Instead, she ends up in a vicious cycle of short-term interventions that either don't help or actively make things worse. The sugar she turns to in order to manage stress increases her blood glucose and her risk of hyperglycaemia. Her bouts of low-carb dieting deprive her gut microbiome of fibre, reducing the production of beneficial SCFAs. And the other casualty is her sense of self-confidence and self-belief. She holds herself back in her life and finds it more difficult to reach her full potential.

PART IV

DEMOLITION – DIETARY DRIVERS OF NEURODEGENERATION

CHAPTER 13

DEMENTIA AND NEURODEGENERATION

I DON'T CONSIDER myself an anxious person. Through a combination of personal experience and professional training, I know that the physical sensations we associate with anxiety are the body's preparation for challenge. If we can learn to understand and tolerate those sensations we can usually overcome most obstacles. I have even been known to draw on nihilism to get myself through a tough time. When all else fails, 'you could be dead tomorrow' does wonders for regaining a sense of perspective. Though I will give angry-looking dogs a wide berth, there isn't much I'm afraid of, not even death. But one thing does terrify me: dementia.

When patients describe spending time with family members with dementia the pain is palpable. They know, of course, that it can't be helped, but it's hard not to feel personally wounded when the grandmother, whom they love so much, can no longer remember them. I support them to bear the anticipatory grief – the grief that is felt before someone dies. With many other illnesses this kind of grief is relatively short: days, weeks or months. But when someone we love is diagnosed with dementia, and begins to decline from it, the anticipatory grief can endure for years.

It is for these reasons – my own terror-induced selfishness and the wish that fewer people go through this kind of hell – that I decided to study brain health (rather than just mental illness) and focus on prevention in mental health. For my nutrition master's degree I reviewed the research literature on nutritional interventions for Alzheimer's disease. How does the food we eat improve or worsen our chances of being struck down by this cruel disease? This is what I present to you in this chapter. But let's start with a brief overview of what dementia is.

Dementia is an umbrella term for conditions causing progressive neurodegeneration and loss of brain functions. These include cognitive functions like memory, comprehension, language and planning, as well as changes in behaviour and mood. As the disease progresses sufferers begin to lose the ability to care for themselves.

Types of Dementia

Type	What's happening in the brain	Early signs and symptoms
Alzheimer's disease (This is the most common type of dementia, accounting for approximately 60% of dementia cases. Women have twice the risk of men.)	Clumps of tangled amyloid protein build-up in the spaces between brain cells, impairing cell signalling. Within the cell another protein called tau takes on an abnormal shape. Tau is required to maintain the normal structure of the cell, so these deformities cause the cell to collapse.	Forgetting recent events, unknowingly retelling the same story, or repeatedly asking the same question. Difficulty finding the right word. Misplacing or losing items. Impaired decision-making.
Vascular dementia	Blood vessels in the brain become damaged or blocked, reducing or cutting off the flow of blood (nutrients, energy and oxygen) to the brain and neurones die.	Poor concentration or comprehension. Impaired planning. Slowed thinking. Mood changes. Unusual behaviour.
Dementia with Lewy bodies	Clumps of a protein called alpha-synuclein (and others) build up within the brain cell, interfering with signalling and causing brain cells to die.	Impaired judgement. Distorted visual perception. Slowed thinking. Problems with language.

Frontotemporal dementia aka Pick's disease or frontal lobe dementia (Less common and more likely to affect people under the age of 65. Often genetically linked.)	Clumps of proteins damage the frontal and temporal lobes at the front and side of the brain.	Distraction and impaired planning. Difficulty generating coherent language. Personality changes.

Since Alzheimer's disease is by far the most common type of dementia, this is the one that I focus on. Throughout this chapter I'll use the terms 'dementia' and 'Alzheimer's disease'/'AD' interchangeably.

At the time of writing, the *Lancet* Commission outlines 12 modifiable risk factors for Alzheimer's disease and other dementias. They are:

- Midlife diabetes
- Midlife hypertension
- Midlife adiposity
- Midlife excessive alcohol intake
- Depression
- Physical inactivity
- Social isolation
- Smoking
- Education
- Hearing loss
- Traumatic brain injury
- Air pollution

Therefore, a third of the modifiable factors associated with increased risk of dementia are *diet/nutrition-related*. There is also a case that depression may, for many, have a dietary component too. Animal studies show a link between the Western-style diet and increased Alzheimer's risk. A long-term HFSS diet increased inflammation in the brains of aging mice and mice engineered to express an Alzheimer's-like illness. The mice also showed astrocytosis, which is an abnormally high number of astrocytes (neuronal support cells). Effectively, the diet made the cells behave as though they were responding to a brain injury.

But even before dementia is diagnosed, dysfunction is evident in a part of the brain that rarely gets the recognition it is due: the blood-brain barrier.

The Blood-Brain Barrier

Your brain is fabulous, but fragile. Just look at the lengths to which the body goes to protect it. Firstly, your brain is almost completely encased in a shell of bone, which is just over half a centimetre thick. There are just a few points of access:

- The eyes – technically a part of the brain. Your eyes are the only parts of your brain to encounter the outside world.
- A few foramen – holes that allow nerves, including the spinal cord, to exit the brain into the peripheral body.

Babies are born not with fully formed complete skulls, but with several bone plates that are held together by fibrous joints called sutures. This configuration allows for some movement during the journey through the birth canal. However, by around the age of two the bone plates will have grown and fused, creating a strong protective covering for the brain. By the time we reach adulthood the skull is surprisingly strong. On average, it takes the equivalent of around 260kg of force to fracture the skull.

So the brain has its very own bone bunker. Not even the heart gets that sort of protection, and the rest of the vital organs are shielded from the outside world with just a little muscle, skin and sinew. Talk about favouritism! But there is another, microscopic but no less important layer of defence. While the skull protects the brain from damage from the outside world, the blood-brain barrier is a layer of specialised cells, tightly held together, that perform three crucial functions:

1. Regulation of brain blood flow
2. Regulation of the transport of oxygen and nutrients from the blood into the brain
3. Removal of waste products from the brain to the bloodstream

If the skull is a crude but effective physical barrier, the BBB is akin to the sophisticated security system in place around parliament: names, security passes, backgrounds and known associates are checked, trouble-makers are escorted off the premises. When the BBB is working properly only the select few (e.g. water and glucose, a few amino acids) make it through. However, a few things can cause the security system to fail. When the integrity of the BBB is compromised the brain inevitably suffers.

A permeable or 'leaky' BBB can allow unwanted or harmful components from the blood into the brain, setting off the brain's internal immune cells and creating neuroinflammation. This brain inflammation is a feature of clinical depression, bipolar disorder, obsessive-compulsive disorder (OCD) and schizophrenia. BBB leakage is seen in mild cognitive impairment (MCI), the age-related decline in cognitive function that is often a precursor of AD. Importantly, BBB leakage in MCI appears *before* the onset of brain cell death and dementia symptoms, suggesting it is a driver of illness progression. Furthermore, BBB disruption is characteristic of Alzheimer's disease.

Clearly a leaky blood-brain barrier is something we would all like to avoid, but what causes it? Physical injuries, like a blow to the head, can, of course, damage the brain and its protective barrier. Similarly, damage to the blood vessels that occurs during a stroke can disrupt barrier function. Low oxygen availability or the presence of infection can also increase BBB permeability. And, central to the thesis of this book, there are a range of nutrition-related factors that affect BBB integrity: adiposity (body fat); diabetes; gut microbiome dysfunction and a lack of fibre; and alcohol.

Body fat

Fat is not an inert storage tissue; it is an active endocrine organ that produces hormones important for health and energy homeostasis. Fat cells also play a role in the immune system as they are able to produce several types of cytokines (immune signalling molecules). Many of these are pro-inflammatory, and one way or another promote BBB permeability. One, TNF-α, promotes insulin resistance and this is one of the reasons that higher body fat is a risk factor for type 2 diabetes.

Diabetes

In the chapter on sugar, we looked at the negative effects of chronically high sugar consumption and diabetes on several features of brain health. Additionally, high blood glucose levels impair BBB integrity through a range of mechanisms, including increased production of free radicals or ROS (those molecules with a troublesome unpartnered electron) by glucose-swamped mitochondria. The ROS accumulate at the BBB, damaging the epithelial cells. Type 2 diabetes, and importantly prediabetes, significantly increases the risk for MCI, vascular dementia and Alzheimer's disease, as we have seen.

Gut

Habitual diets that are low in fibre and high in sugar (like our 55 per cent UPF consumption) impair the brain's ability to protect itself, as we saw in the **Psychobiotics** chapter. Again, this harm accumulates over time, contributing to our worsening mental health and increasing rates of dementia diagnosis.

Alcohol

The metabolism of alcohol increases the production of ROS and weakens tight junctions, both of which impair BBB integrity and function. This is a contributing factor to the known brain harms of excess alcohol consumption.

YOUNG-ONSET DEMENTIA

Dementia is an age-related condition, which means that our risk of being diagnosed with it increases as we get older. However, new research conducted by University College London indicates an increased prevalence of young-onset dementia, where someone is diagnosed between the ages of 30 and 64. Cases have risen from 42,000 in 2014 to 70,800 this year. Though some of this difference may be due to changes in the way estimates are made, the trend has been noted elsewhere in the world too. The rise in YOD tells us that it's not just about aging. Something (or many things) about the way we live is hurting our brains.

Low levels of physical activity, increased air pollution, chronic stress, inadequate sleep, etc., all play a role. But, for me, this vulnerability starts in utero, with the nutritional deficiencies that are common in the population leading to compromised infant brain development. If we are going to reverse this trend, population nutrition – including nutrition education, access and affordability – must be a priority.

Type 3 Diabetes?

I described in the chapter on sugar how chronic elevated blood glucose and insulin (insulin resistance) is a driver of neurodegeneration. Some researchers and health influencers on social media have gone a step further and proposed that Alzheimer's disease is a subtype of diabetes, calling it 'type 3 diabetes'. The rationale for this position is that insulin resistance in the brain is a feature of Alzheimer's disease. However, while there is overlap between the two conditions, unique features of AD mean that, for now, the major health organisations do not recognise AD as a subtype of diabetes.

What is interesting, though, is that omega-3 deficiency can reduce uptake of glucose in brain cells by 30 per cent. Remembering that the brain has a huge energy demand, and depends on glucose, this presents a serious energy crisis for the brain. Impaired glucose uptake in brain cells is associated with poor brain function and neuronal death. Similarly, there is a feedback loop between oxidative stress, dysfunctional glucose metabolism and neuronal death in AD (see page 205).

Crucially, omega-3 fats can both reduce oxidative damage through upregulation of pro-resolving factors (see page 26) and improve glucose metabolism. It is, therefore, likely that our chronically low intakes of omega-3 fats, *throughout our lives*, contributes to accelerated brain aging through long-term energy deprivation and increased oxidative damage. So, it seems we have come full circle; the nutrients that helped to build our brains at the start of life help to protect them in our later years, and the evidence for the protective role of *lifelong* DHA intake is compelling. Let's take a look.

OMEGA-3 INDEX

To test a person's omega-3 levels one method is to simply measure how much of the fatty acid is suspended in the liquid portion of their blood (serum or plasma). However, serum levels are affected by how much omega-3 has been recently consumed. So, if you went for a big sushi lunch the day before the test, your levels might be abnormally high. A more accurate way to measure long-term omega-3 intake is to look at the amount of it that is held in the membranes of red blood cells (RBCs). Recall that though omega-3 fats are highly concentrated in brain cells, they are present in almost all the cells in the body. Since red blood cells circulate for between 90 and 120 days, they can tell researchers about the *average* omega-3 availability during that period. RBC levels also correlate better than serum with the amount of omega-3 in other tissues. So RBC omega-3 (RBC DHA) is a valuable proxy for brain omega-3 levels.

An RBC omega-3 level of 8 per cent is currently considered desirable. Interestingly, this is the same percentage as is found in a healthy neurone. An index of less than 4 per cent is associated with additional health risks.

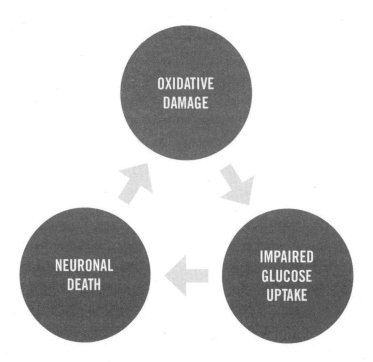

In a study published in the well-respected science journal *Nature*, people with a higher RBC DHA percentage had reduced mortality. The analysis pooled data from 17 studies, which included 42,466 individuals with an average age of 65 and an average follow-up period of 16 years. During that period 37 per cent of the participants died, around 30 per cent from heart disease, 30 per cent from cancer and the remainder from other causes. They found that people with the highest RBC DHA levels (7.55 per cent) had around 13 per cent reduced risk of dying during the follow-up period compared to those with the lowest levels (3.52 per cent). All very interesting, but what about the brain?

By the time someone is in their sixties their brain is shrinking at a rate of between 0.5 and 1 per cent per year. This age-related brain shrinkage is a major factor in the declines in cognitive function that are common in aging adults. The rate of shrinkage is faster in neurodegenerative diseases like AD. In a prospective study of 1,575 older people, those in the lowest quartile of RBC DHA had smaller overall brain volumes. They also had lower scores on tests of visual memory and cognitive function. In an analysis of data from 1,111 postmenopausal women, researchers found a close correlation between RBC DHA and both overall and hippocampal brain volumes. For every 1 standard deviation (a statistical measure of the difference between the individual's score and the group average) increase in RBC DHA status, the women had a 2.1cm³ increase in brain volume. The higher the RBC DHA, the bigger the brain. Knowing that women have twice the risk of Alzheimer's disease compared to men, this feels to me like an important finding. And to highlight the fact that brain resilience starts at the beginning of life, there is also a correlation between RBC DHA, brain weight and rate of brain growth in six-week-old preterm infants. Furthermore, in a similar study of 1,490 people aged over 65, those with the highest RBC DHA (above 6.1 per cent) had a *49 per cent* reduced risk of developing AD compared to those with the lowest (below 3.8 per cent).

What might be happening? A range of things. DHA reduces the brain's amyloid burden in several ways. It both prevents amyloid build-up and facilitates clearance. DHA has been shown to enhance the production of new brain cell connections in the hippocampus and protect against stress-induced damage. Brain scans also show that people with a higher RBC DHA have better perfusion (brain blood flow). Their brains are better fed.

Interventions

So, I have described the studies that show correlations between habitual nutrition and brain health. This is helpful but to be really convinced what we want to see are interventions, studies where a group of people with a condition get a treatment so that we can see whether that treatment makes a difference. Fortunately, we have that.

OmegAD

The omega-3 and Alzheimer's disease study was a randomised, placebo-controlled, double-blind trial of supplementation with 1,700mg of DHA and 600mg of EPA in those with mild to moderate Alzheimer's disease. After six months there was no difference in disease progression between the treatment and placebo groups. This is not too surprising since, as we have seen, it can take several months for fats to be absorbed into cell membranes. However, even in this short period there was a significant protective treatment effect in those with very mild AD, i.e. those at the very earliest stages of illness. Considering that the brain damage that leads to AD begins to accumulate decades before symptoms emerge, I find this very impressive.

The MIND diet

MIND stands for the Mediterranean-DASH Intervention for Neurodegenerative Delay. DASH is Dietary Approaches to Stop Hypertension (a diet designed to reduce blood pressure). MIND combines the Mediterranean diet with DASH to create a diet formulated to protect the brain and slow brain aging. The MIND diet lists ten foods to prioritise and five to limit.

To include:

- Wholegrains – three servings per day
- Leafy green vegetables – at least six servings per week
- Any other vegetable – one serving per day
- Raw unsalted nuts – at least five servings per week
- Beans – at least four times a week
- Berries – at least twice a week
- Poultry – at least twice a week
- Olive oil – as your main oil for cooking and dressing salads
- Fish – at least once a week, ideally oily
- Wine – no more than one glass per day

To limit:

- Butter and margarine – less than one tablespoonful per day
- Red meat – no more than three servings per week
- Cheese – less than once per week
- Pastries and confectionery – no more than four times per week
- Fried/fast foods – less than once a week

In a study of 923 older participants (none of whom had dementia at the start of the study) followed up over an average of four and a half years, the closer people stuck to the diet, the lower their risk of developing Alzheimer's disease. The researchers analysed the results by degree of diet adherence – low, medium or high. Those in the high group had a 53 per cent reduced risk of developing AD compared with the low group. These results were independent of other healthy lifestyle factors like exercise.

Compare the brain-nourishing MIND recommended foods with the average Brit's over 50 per cent UPF diet and you can perhaps start to understand why dementia is our leading cause of death. Encouragingly, MIND has been listed as the easiest diet to follow and even moderate adherence has been shown to protect against cognitive decline.

VITACOG

In this randomised controlled trial researchers compared a daily vitamin supplement containing 0.8mg B9, 0.5mg B12 and 20mg B6 against a placebo. They also looked at the levels of omega-3 in participants' blood (though omega-3 supplements were not used in the study). In the analysis they found something unexpected. In the supplement group only those in the highest tertile of omega-3 intake showed results. So the efficacy of the vitamin B supplements *depended* on baseline omega-3. Only those with adequate omega-3 saw the benefit of vitamin B supplementation. And what were those benefits? A *40 per cent* slowed rate of brain atrophy! Brain shrinkage 40 per cent slower simply from combining B vitamins with omega-3. I hasten to remind you that dementia is our leading cause of death and the disease that adults are most afraid of. And here we have experimental evidence that a cheap and safe nutritional supplement could slow the progression of this devastating illness. Given the repeated failure of anti-Alzheimer's drug research, this is information that we should be shouting from the rooftops.

The FINGER study

The Finnish Geriatric Intervention Study to Prevent Cognitive Impairment and Disability differs from the interventions above as nutrition was one part of a multimodal intervention. But it is well worth mentioning because of its scope and impressive results so far. This two-year study recruited older people (average age 70) who were identified as already being at risk of cognitive decline. That is, their performance on tests of cognition and their heart health risk factors were poorer than would be expected for their age. This kind of mild cognitive impairment is a common precursor of AD. The 1,260 participants were randomised to either receive the full intervention or general health advice. The intervention groups received dietitian-led nutrition advice based on the Finnish nutrition recommendations (see Appendix; NB the Finns recommend eating fish 2–3 times per week), were supported to exercise regularly and engage in cognitive challenges, and encouraged to stay socially active. At the end of the study those in the intervention groups saw maintained *or improved* cognitive performance. This is a big deal. We commonly think of older age as a period of inevitable cognitive decline, but in this group of 70-year-olds who were already at risk of neurodegeneration *their brains got better.* No, we can't put all of these benefits down to nutrition alone but I am fine with that. As I have said, I am not claiming that nutrition is the panacea of brain health, but a gravely underappreciated and overlooked contributing factor. What this study highlights is the importance of moving away from our current 'neck-up vs neck-down' approach to brain and mental health. Improving conditions in the body improves brain outcomes.

MAGNESIUM

Magnesium is one of the most abundant minerals in the body and is required for over 600 enzyme reactions. It plays key roles in a range of biological activities including DNA synthesis and repair, antioxidant production, ATP metabolism and immune function. However, it is also essential for nerve function and health. In fact, the main symptoms of magnesium deficiency are neurological: muscle twitches and weakness, irregular heartbeat, sleep problems, and mood and cognitive disturbance.

Magnesium status decreases as we age because we consume less, it is less well absorbed in the gut and is lost at higher levels in urine. In addition, people with type 2 diabetes may lose magnesium through increased urination. The importance of magnesium for nerve function and the age-related losses have led researchers to question whether magnesium deficiency is implicated in neurodegeneration.

People with Alzheimer's disease have significantly lower magnesium in their cerebral spinal fluid compared to healthy control subjects. Low magnesium in the brain increases oxidative stress, and is linked to higher levels of inflammation in the cells of the blood-brain barrier. In animal studies, low magnesium over successive generations leads to the loss of dopaminergic neurones. Specific to Alzheimer's disease pathology, adequate magnesium can lower inflammation, lower the accumulation of amyloid and improve its clearance, may reduce tau phosphorylation, and prevent synaptic loss. Maintaining adequate levels of dietary magnesium throughout life may, therefore, be neuroprotective.

The richest food sources of the mineral are: nuts (particularly Brazil nuts), seeds, beans, peas and lentils, dark chocolate (over 70 per cent cocoa solids), wholegrains and leafy green vegetables. Though there are concerns about declining soil magnesium levels, if you are eating a wholefood, minimally processed diet you should be able to meet the UK recommended 300mg or 270mg per day for men and women, respectively. However, most people are not eating a minimally processed diet. Instead, they are eating high amounts of UPFs (up to 80 per cent of a food's magnesium content is lost during processing), and not consuming the minimum recommended five-a-day. On top of this, low vitamin D status blocks the absorption of magnesium in the gut and there is evidence of inadequate vitamin D intake in every age group in the UK. Consequently, magnesium deficiency is widespread.

It is not common for people to supplement with magnesium and even if you take a multivitamin and mineral supplement it may not provide enough. Magnesium salts are bulky so they are only included in tiny amounts in multivitamin and mineral supplements. Like choline, though, it is hugely important for neurological health, yet levels in the general population are low.

Overall, the evidence suggests that once Alzheimer's disease has progressed past the point of moderate severity, there is little that can be done to halt or slow the progression of the illness. This highlights the importance of primary prevention and intervention at the very earliest stages of illness. And yes, to be clear, I think prevention starts at conception, when brains are being built. Failing that, the research indicates that the next most important life stage is middle age, at which point metabolic health metrics (blood glucose, blood pressure, waist circumference, etc.) are key risk factors. This does not mean that intervention after middle age is pointless, the FINGER study says otherwise. But there is less return on investment with increasing age.

Despite many billions of dollars being spent on pharmaceutical research and development, the results of Alzheimer's disease drugs trials have, so far, been less than impressive. Certainly less impressive than the outcomes of the nutrition and lifestyle interventions described in this chapter. In her brief time as health secretary, Thérèse Coffey unveiled plans for a £500 million social care fund, to bolster the recruitment of care workers and social care provision. Presumably, she was aware that the social care costs of dementia outweigh those of cancer, heart disease and stroke *combined*. And these costs are set to treble by 2040. Meanwhile, it is estimated that families are currently providing in the region of £13.9 billion of unpaid care every year, with this figure projected to skyrocket to £35.7 billion in the same period. The ripples of this burden will be felt across society: people of working age cutting back on or giving up work to care for parents or partners. The inevitable increase in welfare costs as these people accumulate smaller pensions and eat into their savings. And, of course, the emotional stress of this kind of care is enormous, with unpaid carers often experiencing burnout and depression. Investing in social care in the here-and-now is obviously necessary and welcome, but improving population nutrition, from early life, should be a cornerstone strategy for any government serious about protecting the long-term brain health of its citizens.

A TALE OF TWO BRAINS

Anya was devastated when her *yiayia* died. It was so sudden. She had been well and looking forward to the Christmas holidays before contracting flu, which quickly developed into pneumonia. She died at the age of 85.

Mia's granny Pat's memory had started to fail around the age of 63. At the time she just put it down to not paying enough attention or being distracted, but gradually she began to repeat herself in conversations and have difficulty finding words and remembering names. She was diagnosed with Alzheimer's disease at 65 and died aged 74. Around this time Mia started to worry about the dementia risk for both her mother and herself. She couldn't be sure but she thought her mum was becoming a little forgetful. It was probably the stress of looking after her own mother for years during her illness, but Mia just couldn't shake the feeling that it could be something more sinister. Mia looked online for ways to prevent dementia. She decided to cut back on her drinking (she had got into the habit of having a couple of glasses of wine every night) and to try eating more vegetables and seafood as she read that this could help, though it was going to be hard to change the habits of a lifetime. She was motivated but she did find it a bit of a struggle.

The leading cause of death in the UK is dementia, with an average age of diagnosis of 65 and an average life expectancy after diagnosis of ten years. However, despite having a similar life expectancy, dementia is the seventh leading cause of death in Greece, so assuming that *Yiayia* maintained the same habits and exposures as her country of origin, she would be more likely to die of a respiratory illness than Alzheimer's disease. The damage in the brain associated with symptoms of dementia begin to accumulate 10–20 years before symptoms emerge, namely, in midlife. If Mia takes positive action now she has the opportunity to reduce her own brain health risks.

CHAPTER 14

VEGANISM AND BRAIN HEALTH

ACCORDING TO STATISTICS provided by the Vegan Society the number of vegans in Great Britain quadrupled between 2014 and 2019 to 600,000. Worldwide the UK was the leading source of Google searches pertaining to veganism in 2021, and it is expected that by 2025 a quarter of Brits will be vegetarian or vegan. You may have noticed that many of the key nutrients I have highlighted throughout this book (omega-3s, choline, iodine, etc.) are found predominantly in fish or occasionally animal foods. Does this mean that people who do not consume animal-derived foods are at increased risk of mental health problems? It depends.

Omega-3 Conversion in Vegans

Let's start by looking at DHA, which we know is found ready-made in oily fish and seafood. But before it gets there, DHA starts out as the omega-3 fatty acid ALA, which is synthesised by the chloroplasts in plants (like algae) and is also found in flax seeds (linseeds), walnuts, pumpkin seeds and soybean oil. However, though the biological pathways for the conversion of ALA to EPA and DHA are present in humans, the efficacy of that conversion is very poor. We cannot synthesise as much DHA as our brains need by converting ALA from plant sources. In contrast to how much our brains depend on it, DHA is surprisingly hard for our bodies to make. Furthermore, several factors can interfere with this process.

Firstly, the enzyme pathways that convert ALA to DHA are not exclusive to the omega-3 family. They are shared by the omega-6 fat lino-lenic acid. Found in vegetable oils, nuts and seeds, linolenic acid is the most abundant polyunsaturated fat in the diet. This means that if there is a lot of omega-6 in the diet it can monopolise the pathway, reducing the already limited conversion and availability of DHA. High intake of lino-lenic acid also inhibits the incorporation of EPA and DHA into cell membranes. So even if there is some available it might not be used.

Other factors affecting the ability to convert ALA to EPA and DHA include:

- **Saturated fat** – High intake of saturated fat and trans fats reduces conversion.
- **Nutrient deficiencies** – Vitamins B3 and B6, vitamin C, mag-nesium and zinc are required as part of the conversion pathway. Insufficient amounts of these nutrients can reduce conversion.
- **Insulin** – Elevated blood insulin levels lower conversion.
- **Genes** – Variation in the FADS gene that codes for the desatu-rase enzymes can impair conversion.
- **Oestrogen** – Oestrogen enhances the conversion of ALA to DHA, so women do it a little better than men. But the drop in circulating oestrogen after the menopause reduces women's rate of conversion.
- **Age** – The quality of conversion is impaired with age.

This myriad of influencing factors means that direct consumption of these fats from food sources is essential.

You may have read that conversion of ALA to DHA is upregulated in long-term vegans. However, blood levels still remain lower than in pescatarians, omnivores and vegetarians, and it is not clear whether the increased conversion of ALA to DHA in vegans is enough to supply neurological needs or how long it takes to kick in after an individual stops consuming sources of preformed DHA. Studies that trace the metabolism of fatty acids show that supplementation with ALA leads to an increase in EPA and DPA but not DHA in vegetarians. Vegetarians and vegans, therefore, especially those who are pregnant or breastfeeding, would benefit from supplemental preformed DHA.

Preconception and pregnancy

It is not at all difficult to imagine a scenario in which a teenage girl transitions to a vegetarian or vegan diet unaware of the brain-essential nutrients that are found predominantly in certain animal foods. Should she remain on a poorly planned vegan diet for a number of years her stores of neurologically important nutrients such as EPA, DHA, ARA, B12 and choline will be depleted, as well as important cofactors such as iron, zinc and selenium. Should she later become pregnant, the foetal brain will be supplied with suboptimal nutrition.

The image below is of a brain scan from a 12-month-old baby boy. The pale outer layers (indicated by the white arrows) should not be that thick. Similarly, the pale shape in the middle of the brain should not be that large. This is brain atrophy, areas of brain tissue that have begun to shrink and die.

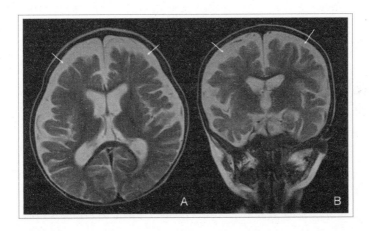

The child presented with muscle weakness, lethargy and smaller head circumference, and made few voluntary movements. This child was not being abused. He was suffering from a severe deficiency of a single nutrient: vitamin B12, having been exclusively breastfed by a mother who had been vegetarian for several years and had not supplemented her diet with vitamin B12. Fortunately, the child responded well to

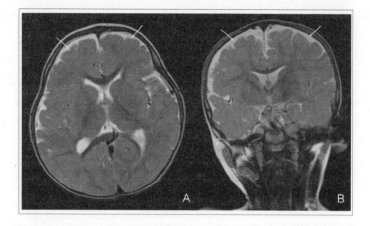

treatment with intramuscular B12, as the second image shows. However, the damage caused to babies' brains by B12 deficiency during pregnancy and lactation is not fully reversible.

This isn't a new phenomenon. There are now over *40* individual case reports from high-income countries of babies as young as two weeks being hospitalised due to B12 deficiency after being born to and breastfed by vegetarian or vegan mothers. These reports stretch back over decades but, importantly, these are the extreme cases. With the rise in popularity of plant-based ways of eating there may be hundreds of thousands of children and adults on unsupplemented vegetarian and vegan diets experiencing the low-level symptoms of B12 deficiency, which include:

- Headaches
- Fatigue
- Pale or yellow skin (in light-skinned individuals)
- Yellow whites of the eyes
- Low mood and depressive symptoms
- Poor concentration and cognitive impairment (brain fog)
- Gastrointestinal pain and dysfunction including diarrhoea, constipation and bloating
- Pins and needles
- Muscular weakness and cramps
- Problems with balance

The problem is that B12 is needed by the body in small amounts so, if someone switches to an animal-free diet, deficiency symptoms may not emerge until 6–24 months later. This can mean that people do not make the link between the shift in their diet and their symptoms.

The case studies mentioned stretch back at least as far as 1981. Over 40 years. And that's the frightening thing: the need for vegans to supplement with B12 is well established. The UK's Vegan Society is clear that: 'It's essential that all vegan diets contain a reliable source of vitamin B12.' Yet babies are still being hospitalised. What about the lesser-known but no less important nutrients that are typically low on vegetarian and vegan diets? Simply, we don't know. It may be that, as with the B12-deficient babies, we will have to wait for enough children to present to healthcare professionals with neurological, cognitive or emotional problems to fully understand the extent and severity of effects.

A diet low on or devoid of animal-derived foods, which is unsupplemented, is likely to be deficient in the key brain-health nutrients:

- Arachidonic acid
- B12
- Choline
- Vitamin D
- DHA and EPA omega-3 fatty acids
- Iodine
- Iron
- Zinc

Although, as noted earlier in this book, choline, vitamin D, omega-3s and iodine are typically low in meat-eaters too. For example, up to 20 per cent of older Brits have marginal B12 status, which is of particular concern given the data on B vitamin deficiency and neurodegeneration. However, those on poorly planned, unsupplemented vegan diets are likely to be even worse off.

Childhood

Again, the rise in veganism is such a recent phenomenon that there is little data on the neurological impacts on children and young people raised on this diet. A recent Finnish study found that, happily, most children on a vegan diet were supplemented with B12 and vitamin D and had good folate intake. However, their DHA, vitamin A and (surprisingly) vitamin D levels were significantly lower than their omnivorous peers.

If there is a relationship between maternal choline and offspring autism risk, we would expect rates to be increasing in the general population, where intake is already insufficient, but a relative increase in risk in children of unsupplemented vegan women. Lecithin, which can be purchased in bulk relatively cheaply, is a good plant-based source of choline. Good plant-based food sources of choline include: soybeans and soy products, beans and lentils, wholegrains, broccoli, Brussels sprouts and peanuts. But, as with fibre, these values are from wholefoods. The information on the choline intake that could be achieved from ready-made and processed foods is not available.

The other (potentially) good news is that a compound called betaine acts in a similar way to choline, so it may be able to compensate for low choline intakes. Betaine is found in wholegrains, beetroot and spinach, providing some valuable options for vegetarians and vegans. However, even less research exists for betaine than it does for choline, so it may be a little while before we have any definitive answers or dietary recommendations.

The nutritional needs of vegan children cannot simply be extrapolated from those of vegan adults. If you wish to raise your child on a vegan diet you must consult a registered health professional for advice on age- and development-appropriate food and nutrition.

Long term

Vegans have a reduced risk of heart disease, which is likely to be linked to generally increased intakes of fruits and vegetables and reduced levels of saturated fat. And while the new adage 'what is good for the heart is good for the brain' is broadly true, in terms of a long-term vegan diet there is one unexpected anomaly. According to a 2019 meta-analysis vegetarians and vegans have a higher risk of haemorrhagic stroke, bleeding in or around the brain. This surprising outcome is thought to be partly attributable to lower circulating levels of B12, vitamin D and omega-3s.

As noted in chapter 3 population levels of iodine are already low in women of childbearing age. If these women then adopt a vegetarian or vegan diet their iodine status will inevitably worsen, with negative effects for their own metabolism as well as the brain development of any future pregnancy.

For many people in the UK and US, dairy is a significant source of iodine. However, too few people know that plant-based 'milk' and dairy alternatives do not naturally contain iodine and other brain-healthy nutrients. On a policy level it would seem prudent to mandate the fortification of plant-based 'milks' and dairy alternatives with iodine, vitamin A and vitamin D. Similarly, vegan meat alternatives should be fortified with B12 and omega-3.

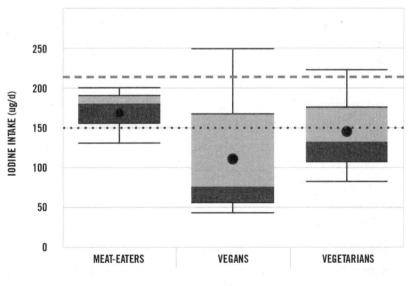

INTAKE OF IODINE PER DIET GROUP

= = = Dashed line is the RDA for pregnant women
· · · · Dotted line represents the RDA for adults

Of course, this is not to say that an omnivorous diet is automatically superior to meat-free ways of eating. As I have described extensively, an omnivorous but highly processed Western-style diet is unlikely to do the brain any favours. Similarly, a vegan diet does not automatically confer benefits on heart health. Chips and Bourbon biscuits are vegan and neither is hailed as a 'health food'. And, of course, vegan 'meats' are by definition highly processed foods. For this reason so-called 'junk food vegans' are unlikely to enjoy the health benefits associated with a 'wholefood vegan' diet.

In general, vegans and vegetarians tend to have lower blood glucose, insulin and lipids than omnivores, bringing benefits to heart health and a reduced risk of some cancers. However, there is no evidence to suggest that a diet free of animal-derived foods is better for mental health. In fact, the trend seems to go in the opposite direction. A recent meta-analysis found that vegan and vegetarian diets are associated with an increased risk of depression. It is possible that some of that increased depression risk is an artefact – women tend to have a higher risk of depression compared to men, and women make up a larger proportion of vegans and vegetarians. However, a combination of common deficiencies in the nutrients that support neurotransmitter synthesis (iron, choline, B12) and cell signalling (DHA, zinc), reduce neuroinflammation (EPA, vitamin D), protect against oxidative stress (arachidonic acid), improve mitochondrial function (B12) is likely to impair the brain's ability to generate good mood.

A vegan lifestyle can be varied, delicious and nutritionally replete when it is well considered. Unfortunately, the public conversation about nutrition and dietary choices too often descends into ideologically driven tribal warfare. The focus becomes proving moral or intellectual authority rather than nutrition. People can and should choose a way of eating that suits their individual biology and ethics. The emphasis should be on providing people with the information they need in order to eat in a way that supports and sustains brain and mental health, particularly when it comes to children and young people.

A TALE OF TWO BRAINS

Around the age of 25, Mia went vegan. She had heard from some of her favourite wellness influencers that it was healthier, would help to clear her skin and give her more energy. She secretly hoped it would help her to lose a few pounds too. These social media accounts assured her that she could get enough iron and protein from a vegan diet, but she read conflicting information about whether vegans needed to take B12 and omega-3. She bought some supplements but only took them sporadically. In the first few weeks she tried hard to make balanced meals (vegetable curries, miso aubergine and tofu, grain bowls) and she felt a bit more energetic. However, it was a big change to make all at once and she soon found herself falling back on vegan versions of the ultra-processed ready meals and take-aways she had eaten before. She was vegan for 19 months before she decided to reintroduce meat into her diet. Mia's experience is pretty typical. Women are nearly four times more likely to be vegan than men and the highest proportion are women aged 18–34. During her time on her rather poorly planned vegan diet, Zoe's choline, iodine, omega-3 and vitamin D status lowered.

Anya flirted briefly with the idea of veganism, but decided she would miss taramasalata too much. She also reasoned that her grandmother had remained healthy her whole life eating a Mediterranean diet that contained fish and a little meat. In fact, she realised she was naturally meat-free 3–4 days of the week. She did not become vegan but she did try to choose sustainable fish and higher-welfare meat when she ate it.

PART V

BUILDING BACK BETTER – LAYING THE NUTRITIONAL FOUNDATIONS FOR HEALTHY BRAINS IN THE FUTURE

CHAPTER 15

THE PSYCHOLOGY OF FOOD CHOICE

OKAY, LET'S SEE where we are. By now you know that the foods we eat have a meaningful and measurable impact on our brain, collective mental health and even our incomes. You have seen that the food a woman eats during pregnancy will shape her baby's brain for better or worse, that hunger is causing some children to be kicked out of school and some adults to be more violent. So, armed with this information, you will just go forth into the world choosing the most nutritious foods and future-proofing your brain health. That's what a rational person would do, after all.

Sadly, of course, it's not that simple. One of my first tasks when working with people with difficult relationships with food is to try to move them away from the belief that food choices are purely rational behaviours. Food choice is deeply irrational. In spite of its surface simplicity, deciding what and how to eat is an enormously complex activity. And the more we understand it, the better chance we have of adjusting the many levers that might allow more of us to make healthful choices for our bodies and brains. In this chapter I present a summary of just some of the many factors affecting individual food choice. I present them in broadly chronological order, so that you may see (a) how the influencing factors layer up over time and (b) that our future eating decisions start to be determined long before we attain the agency or ability to choose.

Preference for Energy-Dense Food

To understand the factors that influence our daily food choices we have to make another quick visit to our ancestral past. Remember that your brain is, metabolically, very expensive; it uses up a disproportionate amount of energy for its size and it is unable to store energy, meaning that it needs a constant, steady supply of glucose. Furthermore, our brain-bodies evolved in environments in which food was scarce, hard to attain (what with all the walking, running, spearing/ catching, digging for tubers, pounding fibrous plants, chewing) and unreliable. Essentially, a lack of food was a big risk for most of our development as a species. For this reason we have an inbuilt preference for energy-dense sweet and fatty food. We find the combination of the two (common in UPFs) even more rewarding.

Biological Preference for Nutrient Indicators – Food Reward

The little bumps on your tongue, called papillae, each contain thousands of receptors for the basic tastes: bitter, sour, umami (which is the rich, savoury taste of meat stocks and mushrooms), salty, sweet and oleogustus. This last one might be less familiar to you as it was only fairly recently added to the canon. It describes the unique taste of fat.

The ability to distinguish these tastes was important because the taste of a food tells us about its nutrient and chemical content. Sweet foods are sources of carbohydrates, and during our evolution it would have been essential to identify these important energy sources. Nerves send their messages using sodium ions from salt, making it essential for the proper functioning of your brain and nervous system. Umami indicates the presence of amino acids, the building blocks of proteins that your brain uses to make neurotransmitters and your body needs to repair tissues. Bitter and sour tastes can indicate the presence of toxins. For example, a class of bitter-tasting compounds called alkaloids have psychoactive or stimulant effects. Nicotine and cocaine are in this group, but so are caffeine and theobromine (found in chocolate). The risk of toxicity or other harmful side effects is thought to be why babies are so much more sensitive to these particular tastes than adults; the bitter taste causes them to refuse and avoid substances that could be harmful. And fat is the most concentrated energy source available, making it very important to survival, especially during lean (and stressful) times.

So, we have a built-in preference (reward) for sweet, salty, umami and fatty tastes, and this bit of evolutionary programming is exploited by food manufacturers, who extract, concentrate and combine these tastes in ways that are unknown in wholefoods. This creates what is known as a 'supernormal' stimulus, one that elicits an enhanced response compared to the norm. In this case, the thing that is being stimulated is your appetite.

But there's more. Salted caramel ice cream with pieces of crisp wafer and chewy chocolate brownie chunks. Here we have a combination of temperature, sweet and salty tastes, and smooth, crisp and chewy textures. Now we are in the realm of 'hedonic escalation' where your liking of the food increases the more you eat it. Food manufacturers invest huge sums of money into research and development for flavour, texture and mouthfeel combinations that will tap into this hedonic response and drive continued eating. But at the end of the second bowl of ice cream you'll tell yourself you were just being greedy.

The composition of the food makes a difference to the likelihood of overconsumption. No one ever complained of an insatiable appetite for turnips. The supernormal composition of ultra-processed foods, high in fat, salt and/or sugar, increases the reward value of the food in a way that can cause our brains to override the satiety signals and keep us eating past the point of comfortable fullness. Now consider that in the UK 55 per cent of an adult's daily energy comes from UPFs and how many times per day food will be prompting a 'keep eating' signal.

In Utero Food Preference

The mother's body isn't just a cosy incubator and a source of fuel for the growing foetus. The mother is the entire universe of experience. For example, as the foetus's auditory apparatus develop, the tone and cadence of the mother's voice, along with the pattern of the vowel sounds that she uses, filter through her body, preparing the foetus's brain for the specific language environment it will be born into. Similarly, tiny molecules of the food the mother eats are present in amniotic fluid. In the third trimester of pregnancy the foetus swallows around a litre of amniotic fluid per day. Tasting and retasting the mother's diet in this way primes the baby for the foods it is likely to encounter after birth. Of course, any notion of choice flies out of the window here. The foetus doesn't even know it exists and its future food choices are already being shaped by what its mother is having for breakfast. A similar process has been identified in breast milk too.

But surely, as the child grows up and becomes more autonomous in their food choices, they can and will create their own eating pattern, right? Probably not. The evidence suggests that our dietary habits are largely stable across our lifespans; the way we eat as children remains the way we eat as adults. This is why we must pay particular attention to the way food is marketed to children.

Programmed for Famine

Like a doomsday cult leader your brain is convinced that the end is nigh. That is to say, that there might be a famine on the horizon (especially if you have experienced severe energy restriction such as extreme diets or food insecurity in the past). So, to ensure that there are sufficient canned goods in the nuclear bunker (fat stores) we have a tendency to capitalise on every food opportunity that arises. You know what I mean. You only finished lunch an hour ago but someone has put a plate of biscuits in the office tea point. Suddenly, and probably unconsciously, you find yourself taking a biscuit or two back to your desk. Essentially, we have brains *programmed for famine* navigating environments of unparalleled, never-before-seen abundance. From this evolutionary perspective, overeating and choosing energy-dense (i.e. ultra-processed) foods is not an aberration, it's not you being 'greedy'; it's your brain doing exactly what it is adapted to do. Like the bodies of the Dutch Hunger cohort – the right behaviour in the wrong setting.

Food manufacturers capitalise on this built-in tendency by placing advertisements for food EVERYWHERE. The more they remind you of the existence of an opportunity to eat, the more likely you are to consume.

The prominence of adverts for brain-unhealthy foods is a policy issue. And not an insurmountable one. From 25 February 2019 ads for HFSS/ultra-processed foods were banned on the whole of the Transport for London network, including all Underground and Overground services, buses, bus stops and roads controlled by TfL, and adverts on roundabouts; taxis, private-hire vehicles and Dial-a-Ride; river services; trams; the Emirates Air Line cable car; and Victoria Coach Station. 'Examples of products that would not be accepted are sugary drinks, cheeseburgers, chocolate bars and salted nuts, while unsalted nuts, raisins and sugar-free drinks would be accepted.' The policy was enacted with 82 per cent support from Londoners, and in the face of hostility from fast-food companies. Some early research indicates that, as a result, Londoners are purchasing 1,000 fewer calories from HFSS foods, a 6.7 per cent decrease. Though further research is warranted to be sure of these results, it fits the established association between advertising, purchase and consumption.

Sensitivity to Food Cues

Another immutable feature of our relationship with the food environment is that some people are biologically (i.e. genetically) more sensitive to food cues than others.

For example, in one study the brain activity in response to images of food was assessed in two groups of children. One group was a healthy weight, and the other group had BMIs in the obese range. The children were shown pictures of a range of foods (e.g. fruit, vegetables, steak, desserts) as well as a range of blurred and non-food images (to distinguish whether their brains were just responding to any old photo). They were presented with the images first when they were hungry and then again after they had eaten a standardised meal. The researchers found that the brains of the obese children showed hyperactivation in response to the food images but less reduction in brain activation *after* they had eaten. Their brains were still excited about food even when they were no longer hungry. Now imagine being that child. You have no idea that this is what is happening in your brain. All you know is that you see food and you want some of it. And if there is nothing stopping you from getting it, then you will eat it. I hope you can see the subtle but important difference here. We are not talking about a 'greedy' child. We are talking about a brain that is *built to be more responsive to food cues in the environment*. There is nothing you can do about the wiring of that individual brain. But what you can influence is the food environment that brain (child) grows up in: the number of advertisements for food they encounter on their way to school or when scrolling on social media, what types of foods are being presented and how appealing they are made to be.

Several other studies have found the same evidence of hyperactivation and a smaller post-prandial (after eating) reduction in activation in a range of brain regions in response to food in adults prone to obesity. The regions identified play key roles in motivation, reward and impulse control. The implication is that people who struggle to maintain a healthy weight have *neurological differences* and enhanced sensitivity to motivational aspects of food cues.

Food Composition and Texture

I mentioned earlier that nutrient-dense foods combining fats and sugars are particularly appealing to our famine-obsessed brains, but there is another feature of UPFs that induces us to eat more: the very fact they are processed. Though it is early days, there is evidence that the very nature of UPFs prompts us to eat more. In an admittedly short, inpatient study (so we must be cautious about interpreting it) US physiologist Kevin Hall's research team compared UPF and whole-food diets matched for calories, sugar, fat, fibre and micronutrients (vitamins and minerals) for 14 days. They found that the people on the UPF diet ate around 500 more calories per day than the less-processed group. When the researchers assessed the levels of hormones in the participants' blood they found that those on the ultra-processed diet secreted less of the appetite-suppressing hormone PYY and more of the hunger hormone ghrelin. Though this perhaps sounds like the same thing, there is a subtle but important difference. It means that the people on the ultra-processed diet felt both hungrier before meals and less satisfied afterwards.

Similarly, a study published in 2022 looked at the impact of food texture on eating rate and energy intake. By definition, the constituent parts of UPFs have been ground, milled, powdered and so on. This means that these foods tend to have a softer texture than their wholefood counterparts (think smooth peanut butter compared to whole peanuts). Because your body uses information from your jaws when you chew to estimate energy intake this could mean that less information gets to the brain. Accordingly, energy intake was highest in the 'soft ultra-processed' condition and lowest in the 'hard minimally processed' group.

Taken together we have the emergence of a vicious cycle: the more UPFs you eat, the more likely you are to overeat. Again, this happens *below the level of conscious awareness*. Rather, increased consumption is an unintended consequence of the interaction of industrialised UPFs and our ancient brain-bodies. On an individual level the solution to this dilemma might be to reduce the quantity of these foods that you purchase. The more your fridge, freezer and cupboards are filled with wholefoods, the less likely you are to overeat. But individuals can't control the food environment outside of their front door.

Supermarket Design

The way your supermarket is laid out is not an accident. I repeat, the way your supermarket is laid out is not an accident. Decades of research have gone into moulding the perfect environment to encourage you to buy more.

- The bright, natural colours of fruits and vegetables at the store entrance put you in a good mood. We spend more when we are in a good mood.

- The enticing smells of freshly baked bread or roast chicken are pumped around the store; a powerful hunger cue.
- Planograms. You might never have heard of these but you encounter one every time you go to the supermarket. A planogram specifies exactly where items should be placed on shelves to increase sales. A key facet of a planogram is 'eye level is buy level'. The region where your eyes naturally rest is where you will find the most expensive, profitable items. You'll find the cheaper products on the lowest shelves. Placing items that are different in nature but which you might eat together are often placed side by side. So you'll find the jars of salsa next to the crisps, instead of with the other tomato-based sauces.
- Impulse buys – cheap snack items – are placed at the till. This capitalises on our innate loss aversion (we hate the feeling of losing out on something), and we'll grab it 'just in case'.
- Volume-based promotions. Supposed deals such as 'buy one get one free' appeal to our inbuilt desire to acquire more energy for less cost. More on these deceptive promotions in the next chapter.

The point is, these tactics work. As we saw earlier, the positioning of products in high-impact spaces in the supermarket is so important that brands are willing to take the government to court to keep their spot. And, crucially, once you have been enticed to buy more, the most likely consequence is that you will eat more.

Stress

Finally, I want to highlight the relationship between stress and food consumption. There is a powerful unconscious shift in food palatability and food choice under conditions of stress. When we are stressed we are prone to turn to sweet and carbohydrate-rich foods to modulate our stress response, and we find these foods tastier and rewarding. I want to note this because, in the wake of the Covid-19 pandemic and with rising social inequality, more Brits than ever are reporting that they are stressed. A 2020 survey reported that 79 per cent of Brits experience work-related stress, 60 per cent financial stress and 48 per cent family concerns. Mental Health Foundation data from 2018 indicates that 74 per cent of UK adults had felt so stressed in the last year that they had felt unable to cope. We already know that chronic stress is corrosive to psychological wellbeing and, as the UK's poverty crisis deepens, its impact on food choices is likely to exacerbate the mental health harms.

This is just an introduction to the complex nature of food choice. However, all of these processes are happening *below the level of conscious awareness*. If your decisions are being shaped by your environment, an environment that itself is the result of decades of marketing and manipulation that prioritises the profits of the food manufacturers over the health of the populace, then have you really been free to choose? And once you had this information, would you make the same decisions?

A TALE OF TWO BRAINS

As we have seen, the dietary patterns that came to govern Anya and Mia's adult food habits were laid down in childhood.

For Anya, it was the regular consumption of minimally processed, simple and home-cooked foods, where the presence of fresh fruits and vegetables was habitual. She grew up seeing her mother and grandmother eat this diet and therefore it was normal for her. These flavours were familiar and reminded her of home and comfort. Her *yiayia*'s distrust of fast food largely stayed with her, so if she did have a takeaway it tended to be a traditional kebab or maybe a pizza.

Mia's first foods were ultra-processed and sweetened, leading to the establishment of a lifelong taste preference for sweetened and packaged foods. She saw her mother eat a limited variety of fresh fruits and vegetables and carried on this family tradition. Mia's familiarity with ultra-processed foods meant that regularly eating takeaways was normal for her.

CHAPTER 16

THE PERSISTENT MYTH OF THE NANNY STATE

ANY CONVERSATION ABOUT reasonable policy precautions to help protect public health is invariably met with vague and shallow invectives about the 'nanny state', a term popularised in British politics by Margaret Thatcher to describe government policies that interfere with personal choice. I can already hear their arguments: that people have the choice to buy and eat nutrient-poor, ultra-processed foods or nutrient-dense wholefoods, as both are available on supermarket shelves. Therefore, it is not the role of a paternalistic government to impose on personal freedom and dictate what individuals choose to put in their own bodies.

However, as we discussed in the last chapter, a combination of genetic factors is constantly driving us to seek out and consume foods with certain qualities. Manufacturers produce and heavily market foods that exploit those innate preferences and vulnerabilities.

So, we can dispense with the claim that food choice is rational and deliberate. What about the idea that government should not intervene in public health? Well, of course, it already does.

Freedom of Choice

Tobacco products are known carcinogens. Cigarettes cause nearly 90 per cent of all lung cancers, as well as cancers of the stomach, liver, kidneys, cervix and more.

Health warnings have been displayed on cigarette packaging in the UK for over 50 years. In 1971 the words 'WARNING by H.M. Government – SMOKING CAN DAMAGE YOUR HEALTH' were added to all cigarette boxes. In subsequent years EU laws increased the specificity and prominence of health warnings on tobacco products, with statements like 'SMOKING KILLS – QUIT NOW' covering at least 30 per cent of the package and additional warnings about dangers to babies and children and risk of impotence covering at least 40 per cent of the pack's surface.

Later, in acknowledgement that advertising and marketing have a powerful influence on the attractiveness of cigarettes, especially to young people, the government sought to reduce tobacco-related harm by banning most cigarette advertising and, by 2017, requiring cigarettes to be sold in plain packaging. The legislation even went as far as listing the specific colour – 'white or Pantone 448 C with a matt finish'. In July 2020 it was reported that cigarette sales had been falling by 20 million per month since the introduction of the packaging legislation and increased taxation.

The key point is that *you can still buy cigarettes if you want to*. You just have to really want to. Smoking hasn't been banned. One's freedom and opportunity to engage in a behaviour that is widely known to be harmful to health has not been curtailed. But now the risks are clearly outlined on the product. The context of the decision has been altered. No, it's not the case that a single cigarette is going to kill you, the damage accumulates over time. In the same way, a single UPF meal isn't going to give you dementia – the damage accumulates over time.

Incentives and the Art of the Nudge

The changes to cigarette packaging are examples of behavioural 'nudges'. 'Nudge' is the term coined by behavioural economists

Richard Thaler and Cass Sunstein to describe how the environment can shape decision-making. Famously, then prime minister David Cameron established the 'Nudge Unit' (formally known as the Behavioural Insights Team) in 2010.

The Institute for Government think-tank explains that: 'People are not the rational economic actors beloved of conventional economic theory – but can be influenced by "choice architecture" into making better choices *in their own interests*' [emphasis mine].

Choice architecture describes the environmental or situational conditions in which a decision is made. It can be as simple as the order in which options are presented or the complex layout of a supermarket. The important thing to know is that *there is no such thing as neutral* when it comes to decision-making. The conditions in which you are making the decision inevitably and unavoidably influence the decision that is made.

This fact means that 'decision architects' (the people with the power to shape environments) have a huge amount of power. And with great power comes great responsibility. Simply, the nature of the food environment influences food choice. So, the question for the government is: is it right that all that power resides in the hands of multinational, profit-driven companies? Is this 'in the interests' of consumers? If humans were fully rational, would they make the same nutritional decisions?

Of course, there is an important discussion to be had about the ethics of unconsciously shaping people's behaviour. I will leave that to the behavioural economists and moral philosophers. For now, I will just deal with the reality. And the reality is that the government do it all the time. So far nudge theory has been used by the government to increase the number of fines and taxes paid, and pension enrolments. This discrepancy makes it seem as though it is fine to nudge when it is in the interests of the government coffers or food manufacturers, but not in the service of individual health. Liz Truss, when briefly prime minister from September to October 2022, ordered a review of the previously agreed plans to improve the food environment – including the 'sugar tax' – under the guise of 'reducing red tape' and to avoid the specious threat of the dreaded 'nanny state'.

Curtailment of Freedom

Allow me to present another analogy. The government's Medicines and Healthcare products Regulatory Agency (MHRA) recommends a limit on the number of painkillers UK consumers can purchase at one time. If retailers are adhering to best-practice guidelines, a shopper will be limited to a maximum of two packets of paracetamol, aspirin or ibuprofen-based products in a single transaction. The products are not banned or only available on prescription, but there is a legislative barrier to access. Why? Because while they are helpful in small doses, they are recognised as harmful at higher levels of consumption. In explaining the policy, the MHRA states:

> *This limit is a reasonable balance between meeting a customer's immediate need for pain relief while helping to minimise stockpiling and accidental or impulsive overdose.*

A moral philosopher might argue that, in a society truly committed to self-ownership, one should be free to decide whether to overdose or not. But that is not (for now) the position we have taken. Instead, people who are suicidal or who are otherwise deemed to pose a threat to themselves are counselled, treated and, if necessary, detained to prevent them from acting on those impulses. That is to say, where there is evidence of harm, the attitude adopted is one of prevention and intervention.

I am not suggesting that there should be a limit on the number of packets of biscuits I can buy in my 'big shop'. I am simply pointing out the inconsistency in the ideological position. When a substance is understood to be injurious at a specific dose, policy is enacted to limit access in order to lessen the potential for harm.

Helpfully, the recommendations go further:

> **Offers:** *Promotional offers on medicines for pain relief should not directly encourage the purchase of more than one pack.*

Explanation: Multi-buy offers such as 'buy one get one free' or 'buy 2 for £xx' may encourage consumers to purchase more packs than they currently need. The customer may stockpile excess packs, which pose a danger for accidental or impulsive overdose.

So, the government understands that BOGOF offers *encourage shoppers to buy more than they need*. It acknowledges and accepts that marketing has a significant impact on our likelihood of buying cigarettes. Yet somehow this isn't considered a concern in relation to food because food is believed to be benign (notwithstanding the 'stockpiling' of energy in the form of body fat).

My argument is that, when it comes to brain health, food isn't benign. Some dietary patterns are protective and others, such as the Western diet's high levels of UPFs, have been shown to be harmful. The difference is that, as opposed to drugs, the effects of food are cumulative, they build up over time, but that does not make the impact any less meaningful. In this book you have seen how food:

- Shapes a baby's brain
- Turns your genes on and off
- Improves or worsens depression
- Influences violence and aggression
- Contributes to the UK's leading cause of death, dementia

Now tell me, if you heard that there was a drug in circulation that could do all of these things, do you think the government would have an interest in its accessibility? As I have shown, the answer is yes. Can you see the incongruity here? It's fine to introduce legislation that makes a product known to be harmful to health less attractive. It's okay to use covert behavioural tricks to get people to pay more taxes. Banning 'buy one get one free' promotions is sensible to reduce the risk of the overconsumption of a substance that can be damaging in excess. But when it comes to foods that have been repeatedly linked to worse brain and mental health *across the lifespan*, such interventions are nannying?

What about the concern that people might be harmed by or simply won't like being nudged to make healthier food choices? Is there evidence to support this? Actually, the opposite. In a paper published in 2020, Dutch researchers used nudge techniques to increase the attractiveness of healthy foods in the canteens of two football clubs. They found, not only that the nudges increased the sales of the healthier products but that, when asked, 78 per cent of participants agreed that such nudges were acceptable.

The Nanny State Is a Myth

There is a long history of, in particular, Conservative governments rejecting calls for public health reform. In fact, from the very inception of public health policy itself. Sir Edwin Chadwick's nineteenth-century *Report on the Sanitary Condition of the Labouring Population of Great Britain* concluded that 'there is an urgent need to improve the living conditions of the poor' to improve their health and, ultimately, productivity. He recommended ensuring that everyone have access to clean water and improved sanitation. Despite commissioning the report, the Conservative government of the time was not keen on intervention (or spending money on the poor). A letter to *The Times* newspaper neatly sums up the general sentiment:

> *We prefer to take our chance with cholera than be bullied into health. There is nothing a man hates so much as being cleansed against his will or having his floor swept, his hall whitewashed, his dung heaps cleared away.*

Subsequently, the Public Health Act, which emerged from Chadwick's report, was not passed until 1948 when the Liberal Lord John Russell was in power.

The introduction of legislation to make wearing a seatbelt compulsory in the UK was derided at the time as 'yet another state narrowing of individual freedom and individual responsibility' by Conservative MP Baron Balfour of Inchrye. In fact, the legislation was officially opposed by the Conservative Party, taking at least ten attempts before it was passed. Within a year of becoming law, front-seat fatalities were down 29 per cent. In excess of 50,000 UK lives have been saved by this bit of nannying. How many more lives could have been saved if the government had acted sooner?

A few years ago, the sugar tax was described by Conservative minister Will Quince as 'the nanny state at its worst'. You can, of course, still buy beverages with sugar in them. The choice still exists but the population-level harm has been reduced. As a result of the levy, sugar consumption has reduced while the number of drinks sold has remained the same. This is a triple win for the government: the public are consuming less sugar, manufacturers have seen no reduction in revenue, but the government has collected over £1 billion in tax income, showing that such policies can improve health and generate revenue. But with reassuring predictability, during her campaign to replace Boris Johnson as leader of the Conservative Party, Liz Truss resurrected the zombie notion of the nanny state. A few years earlier, in an article published in 2019 (nearly ten years after the formation of the Cameron-led Nudge Unit), she wrote:

> *There seems to be an army of nannies and naysayers desperate to tell us we are eating the wrong thing or too much . . . there are calls to regulate or ban foods too high in sugar or fat, to reduce obesity. But people aren't machines – they are agents of their own destiny.*

Not only is this wrong but it is also a glaring contradiction at the heart of Conservative policy. When it comes to paying taxes and fines, people are shaped by their environments. But when it comes to food choices, suddenly we are rational agents. The latter, as we have seen, is more of an ideological position than an evidence-based one. And it is an ideology that is suffuse with cruelty and judgement.

In 2008, when he was then leader of the opposition, Conservative MP (later prime minister) David Cameron gave a speech in Glasgow East (one of the poorest regions in the UK) in which he explained that, 'Of course, circumstances – where you are born, your neighbourhood, your school, and the choices your parents make – have a huge impact. But social problems are often the consequence of the choices that people make.'

In 2013, when questioned by Labour MP Luciana Berger about food banks handing out school uniform, then Education Secretary Michael Gove (currently Secretary of State for Levelling Up, Housing and Communities) responded, 'I appreciate that there are families who do face considerable pressures. It's often as a result of some decisions that have been taken by those families which mean that they're not best able to manage their finances.'

In 2014, during a conversation on BBC Radio Stoke, again in the topic of food banks, former Conservative MP Edwina Currie remarked, 'I get very, very troubled at the number of people who are using food banks who think that it's fine to pay to feed their dog ... but they never learn to cook, they never learn to manage and the moment they've got a bit of spare cash they're off getting another tattoo.'

Now, I am not averse to a little personal responsibility. In my work with clients it is my obligation to help them to understand both what has been done to them *and* what they do to themselves. However, this ideological fixation on the predominance of *choice* in determining one's economic status ignores the evidence of social factors. In 2022, global investment bank Goldman Sachs published research showing that 'compared with other countries, the most disadvantaged in the UK are less likely to climb the income ladder and the economically advantaged tend to stay at the top. Covid-19 has increased inequality further, and recent rises in inflation, especially energy costs, are intensifying the problem'. Their Chief UK economist, Steffan Ball, said:

> *If you look at the UK and compare it with other developed countries, it stands near the bottom of the international league table for both social mobility and inequality ... On social mobility, political debate is often focused on who climbs up the social ladder and that is critical. But it should also consider whether better off families retain their social and economic position. And on this metric too, the poorest and the richest in the UK are the most socially immobile. So this exacerbates social inequalities. Only the US and Switzerland have lower social mobility than the UK.*

Co-author of the research Sharon Bell adds, 'The primary thing is that the UK, relative to the rest of Europe, looks pretty poor on most metrics on social mobility and things have actually deteriorated further in the last few years. So the UK scores very poorly on most social mobility metrics and the key takeaway from our report is that there are things governments, policymakers and corporations can do to help address the problem.' The solution, she explains, is better policy, not better individual choices. When an international investment bank, which exists to serve the needs of the ultra-wealthy, is raising the alarm on the harms of widening income inequality in the UK, the idea that such concerns are solely the preserve of the 'anti-growth coalition' disintegrate into absurdity.

When the poorest fifth of households in the UK would have to spend 47 per cent of their disposable income to achieve a healthy diet, amidst rising fuel and energy costs and record inflation, the only 'choice' currently available is to cut back on more expensive perishable foods. And this is exactly what is happening. According to recent data from the Food Foundation 58 per cent of food-insecure households have cut back on fresh fruit purchases, 47 per cent have cut back on buying vegetables. It is not that poor people make 'bad choices'. Poverty takes away your freedom to choose.

The Marmot report showed us how cuts to government spending were the driving factor behind our widening health inequality, and how austerity measures disproportionately impact those on lower incomes. With the 'cost of living squeeze' already forcing people to make less healthy (but more affordable) choices, you would hope that the government would be keen to put additional safeguards in place. However, I am not optimistic. Not only was the new prime minister, Rishi Sunak, recorded telling Conservative Party members in affluent Royal Tunbridge Wells that, 'we inherited a bunch of formulas from the Labour Party that shoved all the funding into deprived urban areas and that needed to be undone. I started the work of undoing that', but his Chancellor, Jeremy Hunt, has already intimated that pain is ahead as the government reportedly intend to make £50 billion in spending cuts. Should this happen, we can expect the already vast gap in health outcomes and life expectancy between the rich and the poor to widen even further.

Finally, the idea that the UK is anywhere close to being a nanny state is utterly laughable. We are one of the most unequal nations in Europe. There is a housing crisis because the rate of multiple home ownership has increased by 30 per cent since the year 2000. The combination of Right to Buy schemes and buy-to-let mortgages means that social renting has been in decline since 1996. Housing stock has dwindled, permitting small groups of people to build vast property portfolios from former social housing and allowing private landlords to set precipitously high rents. At the same time, we have some of the worst protections for renters. A million more people aged 20–34 were still living with their parents in 2018 compared to 2003 because they could not afford to move. In May 2022 93 per cent of food banks reported increases in demand compared to the year 2019–20, due to the growing poverty crisis. During this period food banks were reporting that people were requesting food that did not need to be cooked because they could not afford the energy. Coincidentally, in July 2022, the owner of British Gas, one of the UK's largest energy suppliers, reported record profits of £134 billion, a whopping five times the profit made during the same period the previous year, a comparatively measly £262 million. Poor people in the UK get sick 20 years younger than rich people and die a decade before them too. Our politicians are talking about pulling out of the European Convention on Human Rights. Even quiet, peaceful protesting now comes with the threat of six months in prison or an *unlimited* fine. At last count (2017) 900,000 people were employed on precarious 'zero-hours contracts' and new legislation has been introduced to make it legal for companies to hire temps and agency staff if their employees go on strike.

So, despite being one of the world's wealthiest economies, millions of our citizens cannot afford to feed themselves or find a safe, affordable place to live. Millions have insecure incomes but limited power to strike for better pay and conditions. And if we protest against any of this we could go to jail. We are certainly, assuredly, at no risk of being nannied.

In his first speech as prime minister, Rishi Sunak promised to deliver his party's manifesto commitments of a stronger NHS, safer streets and levelling up and building the economy. It is a mistake to think that sustainable economic outcomes are achievable with a population suffering under the burden of chronic physical and mental illness, fuelled by a toxic food environment. Nutrition status is lowering UK human capital. But governments rarely see this crucial link.

By now you are well appraised of the wealth of research evidence of this relationship. From birth to old age, diet is influencing brain structure, attention, IQ, depression and dementia risk. Our diets are a health risk. So why can't the government see this?

The thing about food is that it is so familiar. As Yale food historian, Professor Paul Freedman, puts it, 'materiality, necessity and repetition contribute to the apparent banality of food'. Food isn't a microscopic germ or a drug that we might be unwittingly exposed to or whose effects immediately and substantially alter our consciousness. It is leaves and cheese and bread. Boring old oats and milk and ham that we see every day and everywhere. Furthermore, for most of us in wealthy countries there is no limit to how much of it we have access to. In a sense we have become desensitised to the importance and impact of food, which is why policy on its accessibility can be waved off as 'nannying'.

This isn't about overzealous, finger-wagging do-gooders getting a kick out of telling people not to eat chocolate and to suggest otherwise is frankly a slap in the face to committed, hard-working public health nutritionists. I don't know about you, but, personally, I would not prefer to take my chance with cholera or any of the other diseases that can be meaningfully reduced with sensible health policy. But the notion of the 'nanny state' is unleased whenever a politician wants to shut down and disregard reasonable discussion about public health issues like sewers and seatbelts. At some point, the unwavering commitment to a non-interventionist ideology that has been shown to be unfit for purpose time and time again stops looking like 'bold leadership' and starts to look like a lack of imagination or, worse, the inability to update your beliefs in the face of new evidence. In the business, we call that 'belief perseverance'. Elsewhere it is known as fanaticism.

The term 'nanny state' itself conjures the image of a terse, Victorian nanny who raps you over the knuckles with a wooden ruler when you reach for a fondant fancy. But that shouldn't be the first thing that springs to mind when we think of care. Rather, it should be someone who is invested in both your autonomy and your wellbeing. Someone who takes their duty of care responsibilities seriously.

British politics has a lot of problems. Being too caring is not one of them.

Under Construction: Where Do We Go from Here?

Lest I be accused of only raising problems and not solutions, allow me to offer a few ideas. Actually, not ideas, action points. Because just talking about change doesn't create change. The years-long 'conversation about mental health' hasn't improved psychological wellbeing. We need action.

Ultimately, I think Jenny Rosborough, the consultant public health nutritionist we met in chapter 7, was right. Individual changes will not cut it; the adjustments will be too disparate, sporadic and short-lived. Education alone cannot achieve population-level change because changing one's habitual food behaviours takes considerable time and effort. Evidence suggests that, while education is effective at changing a person's *intention*, it has a much smaller effect on *behaviour*. In fact, research published in 2021 by innovation charity Nesta highlights the misconceptions around what interventions are effective at improving public health. In the case of obesity, interventions targeted at the individuals – such as providing education, referral to weight management programmes and provision of digital weight loss tools – are *perceived* to be the most effective. However, the *exact opposite* is true. These are the least effective means of reducing obesity. What works best? Food reformulation, limiting unhealthy food in neighbourhoods, limiting advertising, banning the promotion of unhealthy foods, restricting portion sizes, and taxation. That is to say improving the food environment, using nudges, incentives and choice architecture to make it easier for people to make healthier choices.

What we need is a cultural shift, and that, like the introduction of seatbelt legislation, comes from policy. What we need is a truly bold, forward-thinking, rational government that can see the link between food and mental health across the lifespan. We need a government that is willing to put the long-term future of the country ahead to their own hunger for power.

Cross-party alliances

Any psychologist or behavioural change expert can tell you that, when it comes to making lasting change, the most important factor is consistency. Lasting change is incremental change, and incremental change needs time to accumulate. In this regard modern politics is anathema to lasting change. Politicians on all sides put forward shouty, populist manifestos designed only with the next four years (the length of an election cycle) in mind. What we need are more brave and honest ministers to look across the house to agree to support and implement long-term policies that are in the public interest.

Updated policy on nutritional recommendations during pregnancy

We actually have terrifyingly little information on the basic micronutrient requirements for both mother and baby during pregnancy. Since gestation is a time of rapid brain development, with limited opportunity to influence brain structure later in life, this is an area deserving of urgent research investment, so that we can better advise health professionals and the public.

Improved public awareness of the importance of pre-pregnancy health and nutrition

In the UK there is evidence of wide-scale poor health before pregnancy. While many people are aware there are certain foods that are especially helpful or harmful during pregnancy, awareness of the importance of preconception nutrition is low. When women are having their IUD/ implants removed in preparation to conceive, they should be given preconception health and nutrition advice. Planning and preparing to have a healthy pregnancy should become a normal part of life.

Healthcare professionals wanting to learn more about how to talk to patients about preconception care can find research and resources from the UK Preconception Partnership at www.ukpreconception-partnership.co.uk.

If you are planning to conceive in the next 12 months, head to www.tommys.org/pregnancy-information/planning-pregnancy/ planning-for-pregnancy-tool.

Reformulation of pregnancy supplements or changes to packaging

Most UK pregnancy vitamins do not contain the Cochrane-recommended amounts of DHA or any choline. Women who take these supplements do so in the belief that they are supplying everything the developing foetus needs. Either these products should be reformulated to include/increase these key nutrients, or it should be stated clearly on the packaging that they are missing and need to be acquired elsewhere in the diet. Special consideration of the supplemental requirements for vegetarians and vegans preconception and during pregnancy and lactation is also warranted.

Prescription maternal supplementation

The risk of leaving nutrient provision to supplement companies and individual consumers is that it does nothing to reduce the inequality of access. Wealthier consumers are more likely to be those who purchase these products. This disparity could be circumvented by simply having a programme of free supplementation for all pregnant women. This could be funded with sugar tax revenue. Any additional outlay is likely to be recouped over time in reduced premature delivery (and associated complications), and enhanced cognitive outcomes in future generations (increased human capital and GDP).

Improved public education on the links between nutrition and the brain

The media is awash with health gurus (both qualified and amateur) ready to give us information on what to eat and how to exercise for weight loss, muscle definition and illness risk reduction. But what about the brain? Out of sight and out of mind, the poor old brain doesn't get a look in. An official campaign of health programming would raise public awareness of the links between lifestyle and brain and mental health.

Implementation of the children's health/obesity strategy

The policy is there, ready to go. Now the government just has to do it.

Improvements to institutional nutrition

Having dispelled the notion of 'free choice' when it comes to food, there are some environments where we don't have even theoretical choice over what we eat: schools, hospitals (including mental health facilities) and prisons. The shared goal of these institutions is improvement, whether that is through learning and social development, recovery or rehabilitation. Improved nutrition is a key factor in each case. But here, again, we see wealth disparities. Many private nurseries, primary, prep and secondary schools have professional chefs and restaurant-quality facilities, preparing nutritious meals for the children using fresh ingredients. In contrast, I have visited state schools that don't even have on-site kitchens.

Funding should be provided to permit all schools to produce fresh, high-quality, nutrient-dense meals on site. Some of the cost to the schools of providing those meals could be offset by establishing partnerships between schools and supermarkets. At least 100,000 tonnes of edible food is wasted from food manufacturers and supermarkets every year. This equates to some 250 million meals. (This fact alone, that 250 million meals are going into the bin when there are children in the UK going hungry, should be a source of deep national shame. Child hunger isn't a production problem. It's a distribution problem. It's a policy problem). All of the UK's major supermarkets have committed to halving their food waste by 2030. Incidentally, this is in response to the UN Sustainable Development Goal 12 – 'Responsible consumption and production'. By redistributing healthy ingredients to schools that would otherwise be binned, we could also work towards Goals 2 (zero hunger), 3 (good health and wellbeing) and 10 (reduced inequality). How's that for efficiency?

At the very least, the Ministry of Justice should act on the outcomes of the prison studies and provide micronutrient supplements to prisoners. The evidence suggests that this one change could lead to improvements (and savings) in all areas of the prison environment.

Tax the (nutrient) poor, subsidise the (nutrient) rich

The levy on plastic carrier bags in Northern Ireland raised more than £37 million for environmental projects. Between October 2015 and May 2021 over £180 million was collected in revenue in England. Furthermore, during that period the number of single-use plastic bags dropped by over 95 per cent. The Soft Drinks Industry Levy (aka the 'sugar tax') has brought in close to £1 billion since its introduction (a figure that, by the way, could have easily covered the cost of the voted-down meal vouchers). Similar legislation, a levy on nutritionally poor UPFs, could lead to revenue that could fund subsidised nutritionally rich fruits, vegetables and other minimally processed foods, or a maternal supplementation programme, while encouraging the reformulation of industrially produced foods.

Investment in marine agriculture

What is clear is that our brains require an adequate and stable supply of DHA throughout the lifespan. What is not clear is how this is going to be supplied to the billions of brains on the planet. Fish stocks around the world are at risk from overfishing and habitat decline. We must invest in the means of making increased consumption environmentally sound and sustainable. Marine agriculture may be a good way of achieving this. The production and affordability of plant-based DHA sources should also be considered. It is likely that DHA from industrial microalgae production will be needed to fill the dietary gap. It may be that food manufacturers will begin to fortify more products with DHA as consumers grow increasingly aware of the essentiality of this nutrient. However, the production costs might mean that fortified consumer products are more expensive than conventional formulations, making it likely that those on lower incomes will find a diet that is better for their brain health less affordable. Safeguards should be put in place to ensure that those on lower incomes are not priced out of neurological health.

Mandatory reformulation

It is vanishingly unlikely that we will return to a nutritional utopia where we're bartering our own hand-churned butter for one of the neighbour's artisan loaves. While I think there is great value in encouraging people to eat more fresh foods, education won't achieve the outcomes we need. But policy could be enacted to make ultra-processed foods more nutrient-dense. Flour fortification, minimum fibre content, addition of omega-3s in key foods, for example. Let's make the foods that most people are already eating more nutritious.

CONCLUSION

OUR BRAINS ARE in trouble.

Rates of mental illness and neurodegenerative disease are on the rise and IQ is in decline. There are critical periods of neurodevelopment, during which it is essential to provide key and irreplaceable nutrients. Many of these are in the earliest stages of life. After these windows close, improved nutrition and/or supplementation may be beneficial but they are very unlikely to recoup all of the losses. Imagine a building that has been constructed on poor foundations. You could double-glaze the windows and reinforce the walls but the underlying vulnerability at the heart of the structure would persist.

I am not suggesting that nutrition is the sole cure and cause of psychological distress and mental illness. Social isolation, abuse, insecure work and housing, money worries, genetic risks and more all play their part. But what I hope to have shown you is the unseen contribution of food and nutrition to this overall risk.

And these risks accumulate. Starting perhaps with insufficient brain-building omega-3s and choline during pregnancy, progressing to exposure to sugar-sweetened beverages during adolescence and to insufficient fibre and excess alcohol in early adulthood. Rather than absorbing one short, sharp shock our brains' structural integrity and ability to function well is slowly eroded. We neglect the nutritional needs of our brains. As a consequence, we demand more and more from them ('be more productive', 'be happy', 'be social') while providing them with less and less.

Furthermore, gross disparities exist in the availability and accessibility of healthy foods, with measurable negative effects on brain health across society. According to the Food and Agriculture Organization of the United Nations' Rome Declaration on World Food Security: 'Food security exists when all people, at all times, have physical and economic access to sufficient, safe and nutritious food to meet their dietary needs and food preferences for an active and healthy life.' More recently, in September 2015, the UK was one of the nations that signed up to the UN Sustainable Development Goals, a series of 17 goals with 169 related targets described as 'an urgent call for action by all countries – developed and developing – in a global partnership' that 'recognize that ending poverty and other deprivations must go hand in hand with strategies that improve health and education, reduce inequality, and spur economic growth'.

Additionally, the United Nations (UN) designated the period 2016–25 as the 'Decade of Action on Nutrition' (aka the Nutrition Decade). Member states, of which the UK is one, committed to a series of health targets aimed at reducing the global incidence of non-communicable diseases (cardiovascular disease, cancer, chronic lung diseases and diabetes) and ending all forms of hunger and malnutrition, including undernutrition, micronutrient deficiencies, overweight and obesity. One of the indicators for these targets is the establishment of 'policies to reduce the impact on children of marketing of foods and non-alcoholic beverages high in saturated fats, trans fatty acids, free sugars, or salt' (which is exactly what the obesity strategy was designed to do). In the UK, technically, it is 'delayed pending the decisions of the new post-Truss administration' but given that the most recent health secretary, Steve Barclay, will reportedly be pursuing efficiencies and savings rather than increasing investment in the NHS, the implementation of this policy seems unlikely. Indeed, in December 2022, Rishi Sunak's government delayed the implementation of the proposed advertising restrictions by a further two years.

The Covid-19 pandemic impeded and in some places reversed

progress on many of these goals. But that simply means we should reaffirm our commitment to them now that we seem to be coming out the other side of it. Improving nutrition, particularly during pregnancy, childhood and adolescence, can meaningfully promote progress on these goals.

Decision Architects, Blueprints for Improvement

The government's (eventual) response to the coronavirus pandemic demonstrated that where there's political will there's policy way. Once the urgency of the threat was recognised and accepted, legislation was enacted to reduce the spread of the virus and the risk it posed to the most vulnerable. We went from packed nightclubs and bustling offices to home workouts and back-to-back Zoom calls overnight. Now, here we are with another significant threat not just to our health, but to the very organ that distinguishes us as a species, our brains. If we do not act now the consequences will only worsen. We will see more children diagnosed with developmental difficulties that might have been significantly reduced (if not avoided). Population mental health will erode to a degree that overwhelms health services that are already decimated by the mass departure of burned-out workers. And we will experience deepening inequality in what is already one of the most unequal economies of any developed nation. That inequality itself increases mental ill health. Nutrition deficiency-driven poorer brain development will keep those on low incomes trapped in a cycle of poverty, where ultra-cheap, ultra-processed, nutritionally depleted foods will be the only viable options for pregnant women, children and families. Meanwhile, the wealthy will benefit from a nutritionally adequate but more expensive diet. The downstream ramifications of greater social inequality should be a pressing concern for any government truly committed to the long-term welfare of its citizens rather than just its own desire for uninterrupted power.

We know for sure that a focus on 'individual choice' is insufficient and ineffective for a hazard of this complexity and magnitude, and no amount of ideological wishful thinking is going to change that. Instead, if we want to turn the tanker of degrading population brain health around, we have to think about the *context* in which those individual 'choices' are made. This requires addressing methods of food production that strip foods of their nutrients, and improving food education and the food environment so that people are more able and inclined to purchase nutritious foods, and have the means and opportunity to make nutritious meals for themselves and their loved ones. We really can't afford not to. Mental illness is the single largest cause of disease burden in the UK. In 2003 brain disorders cost the UK economy £77 billion. That figure has since risen to £118 billion, about 5 per cent of UK GDP, mostly in lost productivity.

Any government that has access to this information and then sits on it, doing nothing, is, in my opinion, negligent. Any government that has access to this information and does nothing with it while at the same time paying lip service to 'investing in mental health' is manifestly hypocritical. How dare they? How dare they allow private food industry lobbyists to dictate public health policy? How dare they renege on policy promises that would improve children's health because it doesn't suit their personal political ideology? How dare they think they will get away with it?

With enough people power, we can start turning the tide right now. We can increase awareness among our friends, family, colleagues and social media audiences. And we can demand more from our public servants. And we should. We must.

While today is the endpoint of the past, it is the blueprint, the foundation, of the future. Each one of us is an architect, not just of the brains we build for ourselves and our loved ones, but of the future we want to create.

APPENDIX:
SO, WHAT SHOULD I EAT?

Finnish Adult Nutrition Recommendations

Mealtimes and eating habits are to a great extent culturally determined and individual. **You should eat at regular intervals every day**, for example breakfast, lunch and dinner, and one or two snacks if necessary. Regular meals keep your blood glucose levels stable, control the feeling of hunger, support weight management and protect your teeth from decay. They also help you eat in moderation at each meal and reduce the temptation to have extra snacks.

Add more vegetables, legumes, fruit and berries to your diet! You should eat at least **500g, or five to six portions a day**, of vegetables, fruit, berries and mushrooms. One portion means one medium-sized piece of fruit, 100ml of berries or 150ml of salads or grated vegetables. Of this amount, about one-half should consist of berries and fruit and the rest of vegetables. Some of these should be eaten uncooked, while others should be used as ingredients in cooked foods.

Vegetables, berries and fruit contain plenty of fibre, vitamins and minerals as well as other useful compounds. Legume vegetables, or beans, lentils and peas, contain relatively high quantities of protein and serve as a good protein source in the diet for both vegetarians and non-vegetarians. Plant-based protein is also an environmentally friendly choice.

You should eat fish two to three times a week, using a variety of different species in turn. Fish is an excellent source of protein, polyunsaturated fats and vitamin D. **Nuts and seeds** are good sources of unsaturated fat. You can have some 30g (two tablespoonfuls) a day, or 200–250g a week, of unsalted nuts that are not covered with sugar or other coatings, almonds and seeds (e.g. sunflower, sesame and pumpkin seeds, and pine nuts).

Wholegrain cereal products contain less energy than foods made from white flour. Wholegrain products are rich in fibre and more nutrient-dense than refined grains. The recommended daily intake of cereal products is some six portions for women and nine for men. At least one-half of this amount should be wholegrain cereals. A portion means 100ml of cooked wholegrain pasta, barley or rice or some other wholegrain side dish, or one slice of bread. A bowl of porridge, for example, equals two portions.

Your weekly intake of meat products and red meat should not exceed 500g. This amount refers to cooked foods and corresponds to 700–750g of raw meat. One portion of fish or meat, when cooked, weighs some 100–150g. Poultry meat is low in fat, and poultry fat is better in quality than beef or lamb fat. Meat is high in easily absorbed iron. When eating red meat (beef, lamb and pork), you should select cuts that are as lean as possible, and your meat products should also be as low in salt as possible.

Your need of liquids is individual. It is influenced by such factors as your level of physical activity, the ambient temperature and your age. Most people get enough liquids if they drink when thirsty. The reference intake of all beverages is 1–1.5 litres a day, in addition to liquids contained in foods. You are advised to drink water, mineral water, or milk or buttermilk that contain no more than 1 per cent fat with your meals. You should avoid having sugary drinks regularly, as they are associated with obesity and the risk of developing type 2 diabetes. A high intake of sugary drinks also affects your dental health.

GLOSSARY

Amygdala Two complementary regions of the brain important for novelty and threat detection, memory and decision-making.

Astrocytes Support the development and survival of neurones and can increase the development, strength and activity of synapses. Astrocytes feed neurones by extracting nutrients from the blood as well as being able to produce small amounts of glucose, the preferred form of energy for nerve cells.

Blood-brain barrier (BBB) A highly selective cellular barrier that prevents harmful compounds from crossing from the bloodstream into the brain.

Cerebral spinal fluid A clear, colourless liquid that surrounds and cushions the central nervous system.

Cytokines A group of proteins secreted by immune cells that alert other cells of the immune system and the rest of the body that there is something wrong. When another cell receives this chemical message, it can respond in a range of ways including changing its behaviours and releasing its own cytokines, to pass the message on.

Glia Brain cells that do not send messages but help to protect and support the function of neurones. The subtypes of glia include astrocytes, oligodendrocytes and microglia.

Glymphatic system Predominantly active during sleep, this is the brain's microscopic waste clearance system, responsible for the removal of toxic proteins and other by-products of cellular activity.

Hippocampus Two complementary regions of the brain important for learning, memory consolidation and emotional regulation.

Microglia A key feature of the brain's own immune response. Microglia are able to target pathogens by engulfing them as well as producing powerful chemicals. They also produce cytokines.

Neurone Neurones are the brain's couriers responsible for relaying messages to and from the brain and the body.

Neuroplasticity The brain's ability to reshape in response to experiences. The mechanisms of neuroplasticity underpin brain changes during development and the process of learning and memory throughout life.

Oligodendrocytes Oligodendrocytes produce growth factors, proteins called brain-derived neurotrophic factor (BDNF) and insulin-like growth factor 1 (IGF-1) that promote the growth of new neurones and synapses, and support the survival of neurones that are already present.

Prefrontal cortex (PFC) The front-most part of the brain, which coordinates future and goal-directed behaviours and associated executive functions such as planning, impulse control, working memory and emotional control.

REFERENCES

Introduction

Care Quality Commission. 2020. Monitoring the Mental Health Act. Retrieved from: https://www.cqc.org.uk/publications/major-report/monitoring-mental-health-act.

Centre for Economic Performance & The London School of Economics and Political Science. 2012. How mental illness loses out in the NHS: A report by The Centre for Economic Performance's Mental Health Policy Group.

Crenna-Jenkins, W. & Hutchinson, J. 2018. Access to children and young people's mental health services.

Cybulski L, Ashcroft DM, Carr MJ, Garg S, Chew-Graham CA, Kapur N, Webb RT. Temporal trends in annual incidence rates for psychiatric disorders and self-harm among children and adolescents in the UK, 2003-2018. BMC Psychiatry. 2021 May 3;21(1):229. doi: 10.1186/s12888-021-03235-w.

Ellingwood, B. 1980, An Investigation of the Miyagi-ken-oki, Japan Earthquake of June 12, 1978 (NBS SP 592), Special Publication (NIST SP), National Institute of Standards and Technology, Gaithersburg, MD, [online], https://doi.org/10.6028/NBS.SP.592 (accessed 9 December 2022).

Fuller, T., Singhvi, A., Gröndahl, M. and Watkins, D. 2019. Buildings Can Be Designed to Withstand Earthquakes. *New York Times.* Retrieved from: https://www.nytimes.com/interactive/2019/06/03/us/earthquake-preparedness-usa-japan.html.

McLachlan G. Treatment resistant depression: what are the options? BMJ 2018; 363 :k5354 doi:10.1136/bmj.k5354.

Mental Health Foundation. 2021. Mental Health in the Covid-19 Pandemic: Recommendations for prevention.

Mind. 2021. Coronavirus: the consequences for mental health The ongoing impact of the coronavirus pandemic on people with mental health problems across England and Wales.

NHS Digital. (2020). Mental Health of Children and Young People in England, 2020: Wave 1 follow up to the 2017 survey. Retrieved from: https://digital.nhs.uk/data-and-information/publications/statistical/mental-health-of-children-and-young-people-in-england/2020-wave-1-follow-up.

NHS Digital. 2021. New statistics released on talking therapies in England. Retrieved from:https://digital.nhs.uk/news/2021/new-statistics-released-on-talking-therapies-in-england.

Nobi (Mino-Owari), 1891. Retrieved from: https://ebrary.net/1987/geography/no713_mino-owari_1891.

Nurses.co.uk. 2019. Mental health problems main cause of sick days for NHS worker. Retrieved from: https://www.nurses.co.uk/blog/mental-health-problems-main-cause-of-sick-days-for-nhs-workers/.

Nydén A, Myrén KJ, Gillberg C. Long-term psychosocial and health economy consequences of ADHD, autism, and reading-writing disorder: a prospective service evaluation project. J Atten Disord. 2008 Sep;12(2):141-8. doi: 10.1177/1087054707306116.

Office for National Statistics. 2019. Sickness absence in the UK labour market: 2018.

Office for National Statistics. October 2022. Monthly mortality analysis, England and Wales. Retrieved from: https://www.ons.gov.uk/peoplepopulationandcommunity/birthsdeathsandmarriages/deaths/datasets/monthlymortalityanalysisenglandandwales.

Office for Statistics Regulation. 2020. Systemic Review Programme Mental Health Statistics in England. https://osr.statisticsauthority.gov.uk/ wp-content/uploads/2020/09/Mental_health_statistics_in_England_report_committeedraftforcomment.pdf.

Ross, R.G., S.K. Hunter, M.C. Hoffman, L. McCarthy, B.M. Chambers, A.J. Law, S. Leonard, G.O. Zerbe, R. Freedman, 'Perinatal Phosphatidylcholine Supplementation and Early Childhood Behavior Problems: Evidence for CHRNA7 Moderation'. *Am J Psychiatry*. 2016 May 1;173(5):509-16. doi: 10.1176/appi.ajp.2015.15091188. Epub 2015 Dec 7. Erratum in: Am J Psychiatry. 2016 Jul 1;173(7):735. PMID: 26651393; PMCID: PMC5892450.

Sickness absence rates of workers in the UK labour market, including number of days lost and reasons for absence. Retrieved from: https://www.ons.gov.uk/employmentandlabourmarket/peopleinwork/labourproductivity/articles/sicknessabsenceinthelabourmarket/2018.

Teshigawara, M. in Architectural Institute of Japan (ed.), Preliminary Reconnaissance Report of the 2011 Tohoku-Chiho Taiheiyo-Oki Earthquake, Geotechnical, Geological and Earthquake Engineering 23, DOI 10.1007/978-4-431-54097-7, Springer Japan 2012.

Wooster E. While We Are Waiting: Experiences of waiting for and receiving psychological therapies on the NHS. We Need to Talk; 2008.

Chapter 2: Reign of the Fat Heads

Bradbury J. Docosahexaenoic acid (DHA): an ancient nutrient for the modern human brain. Nutrients. 2011 May;3(5):529-54. doi: 10.3390/nu3050529.

Chang, Chia-Yu & Ke, Der-Shin & Chen, Jen-Yin. 2009. Essential fatty acids and human brain. Acta neurologica Taiwanica. 18. 231-41.

Crawford, M.A., Bloom, M., Broadhurst, C.L., Schmidt, W.F., Cunnane, S.C., Galli, C., Gehbremeskel, K., Linseisen, F., Lloyd-Smith, J., Parkington, J. 'Evidence for the unique function of docosahexaenoic acid during the evolution of the modern hominid brain'. Lipids. 1999; 34 Suppl: S39-47. doi: 10.1007/BF02562227.

Donahue CJ, Glasser MF, Preuss TM, Rilling JK, Van Essen DC. Quantitative assessment of prefrontal cortex in humans relative to nonhuman primates. Proc Natl Acad Sci U S A. 2018 May 29;115(22):E5183-E5192. doi: 10.1073/pnas.1721653115.

Hu Y, Hu FB, Manson JE. Marine Omega-3 Supplementation and Cardiovascular Disease: An Updated Meta-Analysis of 13 Randomized Controlled Trials Involving 127 477 Participants. J Am Heart Assoc. 2019 Oct;8(19):e013543. doi: 10.1161/JAHA.119.013543.

Kitajka K, Sinclair AJ, Weisinger RS, Weisinger HS, Mathai M, Jayasooriya AP, Halver JE, Puskás LG. Effects of dietary omega-3 polyunsaturated fatty acids on brain gene expression. Proc Natl Acad Sci U S A. 2004 Jul 27;101(30):10931-6. doi: 10.1073/pnas.0402342101.

Madore, C., Leyrolle, Q., Morel, L. et al. Essential omega-3 fatty acids tune microglial phagocytosis of synaptic elements in the mouse developing brain. Nat Commun 11, 6133 (2020). doi.org/10.1038/s41467-020-19861-z.

Roth G. and Dicke U. 'Evolution of the brain and intelligence', *Trends Cognitive Science*. May 2005;9(5): 250-7. doi: 0.1016/j.tics.2005.03.005.

Shellfish.org.com. Mussels. 2010 Retrieved from: http://www.shellfish.org.uk/files/Healthy-Eating/68944SAGB musselsfactsheet final.pdf.

Vedin I, Cederholm T, Freund-Levi Y, Basun H, Garlind A, Irving GF, Eriksdotter-Jönhagen M, Wahlund LO, Dahlman I, Palmblad J. Effects of DHA-rich n-3 fatty acid supplementation on gene expression in blood mononuclear leukocytes: the OmegAD study. PLoS One. 2012;7(4):e35425. doi: 10.1371/journal.pone.0035425.

Zihlman, A.L. and Bolter, D.R. 'Body composition in *Pan paniscus* compared with *Homo sapiens* has implications for changes during human evolution', Proceedings of the National Academy of Sciences of the United States of America. June 2015;112(24): 7466-7471. DOI: 10.1073/pnas.1505071112.

Chapter 3: The Maternal Universe

Adhvaryu, Achyuta R. et al. 'When It Rains It Pours: The Long-Run Economic Impacts of Salt Iodization in the United States'. Review of Economics and Statistics 102 (2020): 395-407.

Bath SC, Steer CD, Golding J, Emmett P, Rayman MP. Effect of inadequate iodine status in UK pregnant women on cognitive outcomes in their children: results from the Avon Longitudinal Study of Parents and Children (ALSPAC). Lancet. 2013 Jul 27;382(9889):331-7. doi: 10.1016/S0140-6736(13)60436-5.

British Dietetic Association. 2019. Iodine: Food fact sheet.

Hibbeln, J.R., J.M. Davis, C. Steer, P. Emmett, I. Rogers, C. Williams, J. Golding. 'Maternal seafood consumption in pregnancy and neurodevelopmental outcomes in childhood (ALSPAC study): an observational cohort study'. *Lancet*. 17 Feb 2007;369(9561):578-85. doi: 10.1016/S0140-6736(07)60277-3. PMID: 17307104.

Joffre C, Rey C, Layé S. N-3 Polyunsaturated Fatty Acids and the Resolution of Neuroinflammation. Front Pharmacol. 2019 Sep 13;10:1022. doi: 10.3389/fphar.2019.01022.

McNulty H, Rollins M, Cassidy T, Caffrey A, Marshall B, Dornan J, McLaughlin M, McNulty BA, Ward M, Strain JJ, Molloy AM, Lees-Murdock DJ, Walsh CP, Pentieva K. Effect of continued folic acid supplementation beyond the first trimester of pregnancy on cognitive performance in the child: a follow-up study from a randomized controlled trial (FASSTT Offspring Trial). BMC Med. 2019 Oct 31;17(1):196. doi: 10.1186/s12916-019-1432-4.

Serrano NC, Quintero-Lesmes DC, Becerra-Bayona S, Guio E, Beltran M, Paez MC, Ortiz R, Saldarriaga W, Diaz LA, Monterrosa Á, Miranda J, Mesa CM, Sanin JE, Monsalve G, Dudbridge F, Hingorani AD, Casas JP. Association of pre-eclampsia risk with maternal levels of folate, homocysteine and vitamin B12 in Colombia: A case-control study. PLoS One. 2018 Dec 6;13(12):e0208137. doi: 10.1371/journal.pone.0208137.

Stephenson J, Heslehurst N, Hall J, Schoenaker DAJM, Hutchinson J, Cade JE, Poston L, Barrett G, Crozier SR, Barker M, Kumaran K, Yajnik CS, Baird J, Mishra GD. Before the beginning: nutrition and lifestyle in the preconception period and its importance for future health. Lancet. 2018 May 5;391(10132):1830-1841. doi: 10.1016/S0140-6736(18)30311-8.

World Health Organisation. 2007. Assessment of iodine deficiency disorders and monitoring their elimination: a guide for programme managers, 3rd ed.

Yuan He, An Pan, Frank B Hu, Xu Ma, 2016. Folic acid supplementation, birth defects, and adverse pregnancy outcomes in Chinese women: a population-based mega-cohort study.

Chapter 4: The Importance of DHA

Bazinet, R. P., & Layé, S. 2014. Polyunsaturated fatty acids and their metabolites in brain function and disease. *Nature Reviews Neuroscience*, 15(12), 771–785. doi:10.1038\nrn3820.

Bratsberg B, Rogeberg O. Flynn effect and its reversal are both environmentally caused. Proc Natl Acad Sci U S A. 2018 Jun 26;115(26):6674-6678. doi: 10.1073/pnas.1718793115.

Cao D, Kevala K, Kim J, Moon HS, Jun SB, Lovinger D, Kim HY. Docosahexaenoic acid promotes hippocampal neuronal development and synaptic function. J Neurochem. 2009 Oct;111(2):510-21. doi: 10.1111/j.1471-4159.2009.06335.x.

Cave C, Hein N, Smith LM, Anderson-Berry A, Richter CK, Bisselou KS, Appiah AK, Kris-Etherton P, Skulas-Ray AC, Thompson M, Nordgren TM, Hanson C, Thoene M. Omega-3 Long-Chain Polyunsaturated Fatty Acids Intake by Ethnicity, Income, and Education Level in the United States: NHANES 2003-2014. Nutrients. 2020 Jul 9;12(7):2045. doi: 10.3390/nu12072045.

Centre for Policy Studies. 2013. The 2013 Margaret Thatcher Lecture - Boris Johnson. Retrieved from: https://cps.org.uk/events/post/2013/the-2013-margaret-thatcher-lecture-boris-johnson/.

Dubois Julien, Galdi Paola, Paul Lynn K. and Adolphs Ralph 2018A distributed brain network predicts general intelligence from resting-state human neuroimaging dataPhil. Trans. R. Soc. doi10.1098/rstb.2017.0284.

Flynn, James & Shayer, Michael. (2018). IQ decline and Piaget: Does the rot start at the top?. Intelligence. 66. 10.1016/j.intell.2017.11.010.

Golding J, Taylor C, Iles-Caven Y, Gregory S. The benefits of fish intake: Results concerning prenatal mercury exposure and child outcomes from the ALSPAC prebirth cohort. Neurotoxicology. 2022 Jul;91:22-30. doi: 10.1016/j.neuro.2022.04.012.

Gould JF, Makrides M, Gibson RA, Sullivan TR, McPhee AJ, Anderson PJ, Best KP, Sharp M, Cheong JLY, Opie GF, Travadi J, Bednarz JM, Davis PG, Simmer K, Doyle LW, Collins CT. Neonatal Docosahexaenoic Acid in Preterm Infants and Intelligence at 5 Years. N Engl J Med. 2022 Oct 27;387(17):1579-1588. doi: 10.1056/NEJMoa2206868.

Krol KM, Grossmann T. Psychological effects of breastfeeding on children and mothers. Bundesgesundheitsblatt Gesundheitsforschung Gesundheitsschutz. 2018 Aug; 61(8):977-985. doi: 10.1007/s00103-018-2769-0.

Middleton P, Gomersall JC, Gould JF, Shepherd E, Olsen SF, Makrides M. Omega-3 fatty acid addition during pregnancy. Cochrane Database of Systematic Reviews 2018, Issue 11. Art. No.: CD003402. DOI: 10.1002/14651858.CD003402.pub3.

Mörelius E, Örtenstrand A, Theodorsson E, Frostell A. A randomised trial of continuous skin-to-skin contact after preterm birth and the effects on salivary cortisol, parental stress, depression, and breastfeeding. Early Hum Dev. 2015 Jan;91(1):63-70. doi: 10.1016/j.earlhumdev.2014.12.005.

National Institute for Health and Care Excellence. 2021. Maternal and child nutrition: nutrition and weight management in pregnant women, and nutrition in children up to 5 years – Final Scope.

National Institute of Health. 2017. What are the risk factors for preterm labor and birth? Retrieved from: https://www.nichd.nih.gov/health/topics/preterm/condition info/who_risk.

NHS Digital. 2019. Maternity Services Monthly Statistics June 2019, experimental statistics. Retrieved from: https://digital.nhs.uk/data-and-information/publications/statistical/maternity-services-monthly-statistics/june-2019/births.

NHS. North Central London Joint Formulary Committee.2019. Guidance for the review of omega-3 fatty acids (including Omacor®). Retrieved from: https://www.ncl-mon.nhs.uk/wp-content/uploads/Guidelines/2_Guidance_for_the_review_of_omega_3_fatty_acids.pdf.

Nosarti C, Reichenberg A, Murray RM, et al. Preterm Birth and Psychiatric Disorders in Young Adult Life. Arch Gen Psychiatry. 2012;69(6):610–617. doi:10.1001/archgenpsychiatry.2011.1374.

Orloff NC, Hormes JM. Pickles and ice cream! Food cravings in pregnancy: hypotheses, preliminary evidence, and directions for future research. Front Psychol. 2014 Sep 23;5:1076. doi: 10.3389/fpsyg.2014.01076.

Patin RV, Vítolo MR, Valverde MA, Carvalho PO, Pastore GM, Lopez FA. The influence of sardine consumption on the omega-3 fatty acid content of mature human milk. J Pediatr (Rio J). 2006 Jan-Feb;82(1):63-9. doi: 10.2223/JPED.1439.

Pietschnig, Jakob & Gittler, Georg. (2015). A reversal of the Flynn effect for spatial perception in German-speaking countries: Evidence from a cross-temporal IRT-based meta-analysis (1977–2014). Intelligence. 53. 145-153. 10.1016/j.intell.2015.10.004.

Products, Nutrition. (2013). Scientific Opinion on nutrient requirements and dietary intakes of infants and young children in the European Union. EFSA Journal. 11. 10.2903/j.efsa.2013.3408.

Sarah U Morton, Rutvi Vyas, Borjan Gagoski, Catherine Vu, Jonathan Litt, Ryan J Larsen, Matthew J Kuchan, John B Lasekan, Brad P Sutton, P Ellen Grant, Yangming Ou, Maternal Dietary Intake of Omega-3 Fatty Acids Correlates Positively with Regional Brain Volumes in 1-Month-Old Term Infants, *Cerebral Cortex*, Volume 30, Issue 4, April 2020, Pages 2057–2069, doi: 10.1093/cercor/bhz222.

Scientific Advisory Committee on Nutrition. 2004. Advice on fish consumption: benefits & risks.

Teasdale, Thomas & Owen, David. (2005). A long-term rise and recent decline in intelligence test performance: The Flynn Effect in reverse. Personality and Individual Differences. 139. 837-843. 10.1016/j.paid.2005.01.029.

The Equality Trust. 2014. The cost of inequality. Retrieved from: https://equality trust.org.uk/resource/cost-inequality.

Wierzejska R, Jarosz M, Wojda B, Siuba-Strzelińska M. Dietary intake of DHA during pregnancy: a significant gap between the actual intake and current nutritional recommendations. Rocz Panstw Zakl Hig. 2018;69(4):381-386. doi: 10.32394/rpzh.2018.0044.

World Health Organisation. 2018. Preterm birth. Retrieved from: https://www.who.int/news-room/fact-sheets/detail/preterm-birth.

World Health Organisation. 2018. New global estimates on preterm birth published. Retrieved from: https://www.who.int/reproductivehealth/global-estimates-preterm-birth/en/.

Zou R, El Marroun H, Voortman T, Hillegers M, White T, Tiemeier H. Maternal polyunsaturated fatty acids during pregnancy and offspring brain development in childhood. Am J Clin Nutr. 2021 Jul 1;114(1):124-133. doi: 10.1093/ajcn/nqab049.

Chapter 5: Choline

Bahnfleth, CL, Strupp, BJ, Caudill, MA, Canfield, RL. Prenatal choline supplementation improves child sustained attention: A 7-year follow-up of a randomized controlled feeding trial. *FASEB J.* 2022; 36:e22054. doi:10.1096/fj.202101217R.

Bonnet-Brilhault F, Rajerison TA, Paillet C, Guimard-Brunault M, Saby A, Ponson L, Tripi G, Malvy J, Roux S. Autism is a prenatal disorder: Evidence from late gestation brain overgrowth. Autism Res. 2018 Dec;11(12):1635-1642. doi: 10.1002/aur.2036.

Kevin C Klatt, Melissa Q McDougall, Olga V Malysheva, Siraphat Taesuwan, Aura (Alex) P Loinard-González, Julie E H Nevins, Kara Beckman, Ruchika Bhawal, Elizabeth Anderson, Sheng Zhang, Erica Bender, Kristina H Jackson, D Janette King, Roger A Dyer, Srisatish Devapatla, Ramesh Vidavalur, J Thomas Brenna, Marie A Caudill, Prenatal choline supplementation improves biomarkers of maternal docosahexaenoic acid (DHA) status among pregnant participants consuming supplemental DHA: a randomized controlled trial, *The American Journal of Clinical Nutrition*, Volume 116, Issue 3, September 2022, Pages 820–832, https://doi.org/10.1093/ajcn/nqac147.

McClelland, M. M., Cameron, C. E., Connor, C. M., Farris, C. L., Jewkes, A. M., & Morrison, F. J. (2007). Links between behavioral regulation and preschoolers' literacy, vocabulary, and math skills. *Developmental Psychology*, 43(4), 947–959. https://doi.org/10.1037/0012-1649.43.4.947.

Metallidou, Panayiota & Malegiannaki, Amaryllis & Konstantinopoulou, Eleni & Kiosseoglou, Grigoris. (2016). Effects of Different Functions of Attention on School Grades in Primary School Children. Journal of Education and Human Development. 5. 68-79.

NHS Healthy Start. 2022. Healthcare professionals. Retrieved from: https://www.healthystart.nhs.uk/healthcare-professionals/.

Olson A, Zhang F, Cao H, Baranova A, Slavin M. *In silico* Gene Set and Pathway Enrichment Analyses Highlight Involvement of Ion Transport in Cholinergic Pathways in Autism: Rationale for Nutritional Intervention. Front Neurosci. 2021 Apr 20;15:648410. doi: 10.3389/fnins.2021.648410.

Perry EK, Lee ML, Martin-Ruiz CM, Court JA, Volsen SG, Merrit J, Folly E, Iversen PE, Bauman ML, Perry RH, Wenk GL. Cholinergic activity in autism: abnormalities in the cerebral cortex and basal forebrain. *Am J Psychiatry*. 2001 Jul;158(7):1058-66. doi: 10.1176/appi.ajp.158.7.1058.

Ramirez-Celis, A., Croen, L.A., Yoshida, C.K. *et al*. Maternal autoantibody profiles as biomarkers for ASD and ASD with co-occurring intellectual disability. *Mol Psychiatry* (2022). https://doi.org/10.1038/s41380-022-01633-4.

Ronald A, Pennell CE, Whitehouse AJ. Prenatal Maternal Stress Associated with ADHD and Autistic Traits in early Childhood. Front Psychol. 2011 Jan 19;1:223. doi: 10.3389/fpsyg.2010.00223.

Rossignol DA, Frye RE. The use of medications approved for Alzheimer's disease in autism spectrum disorder: a systematic review. Front Pediatr. 2014 Aug 22;2:87. doi: 10.3389/fped.2014.00087.

Rothman KJ, Moore LL, Singer MR, Nguyen US, Mannino S, Milunsky A. Teratogenicity of high vitamin A intake. N Engl J Med. 1995 Nov 23;333(21):1369-73. doi: 10.1056/NEJM199511233332101.

The Vegan Society. 2021. 'Changing Diets During the Covid-19 Pandemic'. Retrieved from: https://www.vegansociety.com/sites/default/files/uploads/downloads/Changing Diets During the Covid-19 Pandemic.pdf.

Tioleco N, Silberman AE, Stratigos K, Banerjee-Basu S, Spann MN, Whitaker AH, Turner JB. Prenatal maternal infection and risk for autism in offspring: A meta-analysis. Autism Res. 2021 Jun;14(6):1296-1316. doi: 10.1002/aur.2499.

Vennemann, F., Ioannidou, S., Valsta, L., Dumas, C., Ocké, M., Mensink, G., Héraud, F. (2015). Dietary intake and food sources of choline in European populations. *British Journal of Nutrition, 114*(12), 2046-2055. doi:10.1017/S0007114515003700.

Wallace TC, Blusztajn JK, Caudill MA, Klatt KC, Natker E, Zeisel SH, Zelman KM. Choline: The Underconsumed and Underappreciated Essential Nutrient. Nutr Today. 2018 Nov-Dec;53(6):240-253. doi: 10.1097/NT.0000000000000302.

Chapter 6: Sugar

Aeberli, I., P.A. Gerber, M. Hochuli, S. Kohler, S.R. Haile, I. Gouni-Berthold, H.K. Berthold, G.A. Spinas, K. Berneis. 'Low to moderate sugar-sweetened beverage consumption impairs glucose and lipid metabolism and promotes inflammation in healthy young men: a randomized controlled trial'. *Am J Clin Nutr*. Aug 2011;94(2):479-85. doi: 10.3945/ajcn.111.013540. Epub 2011 Jun 15. PMID: 21677052.

Campbell, D. 2022. Thérèse Coffey scraps promised paper on health inequality. *The Guardian*. Retrieved from: https://www.theguardian.com/politics/2022/sep/29/therese-coffey-scraps-promised-paper-on-health-inequality.

Camprubi Robles M, Campoy C, Garcia Fernandez L, Lopez-Pedrosa JM, Rueda R, Martin MJ. Maternal Diabetes and Cognitive Performance in the Offspring: A Systematic Review and Meta-Analysis. PLoS One. 2015 Nov 13;10(11):e0142583. doi: 10.1371/journal.pone.0142583.

Cohen JFW, Rifas-Shiman SL, Young J, Oken E. Associations of Prenatal and Child Sugar Intake With Child Cognition. Am J Prev Med. 2018 Jun;54(6):727-735. doi: 10.1016/j.amepre.2018.02.020.

Devarshi PP, Grant RW, Ikonte CJ, Hazels Mitmesser S. Maternal Omega-3 Nutrition, Placental Transfer and Fetal Brain Development in Gestational Diabetes and Preeclampsia. Nutrients. 2019 May 18;11(5):1107. doi: 10.3390/nu11051107.

Food Foundation. 2022. The Broken Plate: The State of the Nation's Food System https://foodfoundation.org.uk/sites/default/files/2022-07/FF_BP_AT A GLANCE.pdf.

Fraser A, Nelson SM, Macdonald-Wallis C, Lawlor DA. Associations of existing diabetes, gestational diabetes, and glycosuria with offspring IQ and educational attainment: the Avon Longitudinal Study of Parents and Children. Exp Diabetes Res. 2012;2012: 963735. doi: 10.1155/2012/963735.

Ghosal S, Arora B, Dutta K, Ghosh A, Sinha B, Misra A. Increase in the risk of type 2 diabetes during lockdown for the COVID19 pandemic in India: A cohort analysis. Diabetes Metab Syndr. 2020 Sep-Oct;14(5):949-952. doi: 10.1016/j.dsx.2020.06.020.

H Al Wattar B, Dodds J, Placzek A, Beresford L, Spyreli E, Moore A, Gonzalez Carreras FJ, Austin F, Murugesu N, Roseboom TJ, Bes-Rastrollo M, Hitman GA, Hooper R, Khan KS, Thangaratinam S; ESTEEM study group. Mediterranean-style diet in pregnant women with metabolic risk factors (ESTEEM): A pragmatic multicentre randomised trial. PLoS Med. 2019 Jul 23;16(7):e1002857. doi: 10.1371/journal. pmed.1002857.

Health state life expectancies by national deprivation deciles, England: 2018 to 2020. Retrieved from: https://www.ons.gov.uk/peoplepopulationandcommunity/healthand socialcare/healthinequalities/bulletins/healthstatelifeexpectanciesbyindexofmultiple deprivationimd/latest.

Jacques A, Chaaya N, Beecher K, Ali SA, Belmer A, Bartlett S. The impact of sugar consumption on stress driven, emotional and addictive behaviors. Neurosci Biobehav Rev. 2019 Aug;103:178-199. doi: 10.1016/j.neubiorev.2019.05.021.

Javid, S. 2022. Sajid Javid's resignation speech in full. The *Spectator*. Retrieved from: https://www.spectator.co.uk/article/sajid-javid-s-resignation-speech-in-full.

Kellogg's Frosties Breakfast Cereal 500g. Retrieved from: https://www.sainsburys. co.uk/gol-ui/product/kelloggs-frosties-cereal-500g-2059600-p.

Linda S. Geiss, Yanfeng Li, Israel Hora, Ann Albright, Deborah Rolka, Edward W. Gregg; Resurgence of Diabetes-Related Nontraumatic Lower-Extremity Amputation in the Young and Middle-Aged Adult U.S. Population. *Diabetes Care* 1 January 2019; 42 (1): 50–54. doi 10.2337/dc18-1380.

Lundeen EA, Park S, Onufrak S, Cunningham S, Blanck HM. Adolescent Sugar-Sweetened Beverage Intake is Associated With Parent Intake, Not Knowledge of Health Risks. Am J Health Promot. 2018 Nov;32(8):1661-1670. doi: 10.1177/ 0890117118763008.

Mifsud S, Schembri EL, Gruppetta M. Stress-induced hyperglycaemia. Br J Hosp Med (Lond). 2018 Nov 2;79(11):634-639. doi: 10.12968/hmed.2018.79.11.634.

NHS. 2020. Sugar: The facts. Retrieved from: https://www.nhs.uk/live-well/eat-well/food-types/how-does-sugar-in-our-diet-affect-our-health/.

Office for National Statistics. 2022. Health state life expectancies by national deprivation deciles, England: 2018 to 2020. Retrieved from: https://www.ons.gov.uk/peoplepopu-lationandcommunity/healthandsocialcare/healthinequalities/bulletins/healthstatelifeex-pectanciesbyindexofmultipledeprivationimd/2018to2020.

Office for National Statistics. 2022. Health state life expectancies by national deprivation deciles, England.

O'Mahoney LL, Matu J, Price OJ, Birch KM, Ajjan RA, Farrar D, Tapp R, West DJ, Deighton K, Campbell MD. Omega-3 polyunsaturated fatty acids favourably modulate cardiometabolic biomarkers in type 2 diabetes: a meta-analysis and meta-regression of randomized controlled trials. Cardiovasc Diabetol. 2018 Jul 7;17(1):98. doi: 10.1186/ s12933-018-0740-x.

Paige K Berger, Jasmine F Plows, Roshonda B Jones, Tanya L Alderete, Claudia Rios, Trevor A Pickering, David A Fields, Lars Bode, Bradley S Peterson, Michael I Goran, Associations of maternal fructose and sugar-sweetened beverage and juice intake during lactation with infant neurodevelopmental outcomes at 24 months, *The American Journal of Clinical Nutrition*, Volume 112, Issue 6, December 2020, Pages 1516–1522, doi.10.1093/ajcn/nqaa255.

Pase, M.P., J.J. Himali, P.F. Jacques, C. DeCarli, C.L. Satizabal, H. Aparicio, R.S. Vasan, A.S. Beiser, S. Seshadri. 'Sugary beverage intake and preclinical Alzheimer's disease in the community'. *Alzheimers Dement.* Sep 2017;13(9):955-964. doi: 10.1016/j.jalz.2017.01.024. Epub 2017 Mar 6. PMID: 28274718; PMCID: PMC6820519.

Schmitt JA, Ashraf AP, Becker DJ, Sen B. Changes in Type 2 Diabetes Trends in Children and Adolescents During the COVID-19 Pandemic. J Clin Endocrinol Metab. 2022 Jun 16;107(7):e2777-e2782. doi: 10.1210/clinem/dgac209.

Sherman, G.D. and P.H. Mehta. 'Stress, cortisol, and social hierarchy'. *Curr Opin Psychol.* Jun 2020;33:227-232. doi: 10.1016/j.copsyc.2019.09.013. Epub 2019 Oct 19. PMID: 31765930.

Sweney, M. 2022. Kellogg's to challenge new UK rules for high-sugar cereals in court. https://www.theguardian.com/business/2022/apr/27/kelloggs-court-challenge-new-uk-rules-high-sugar-cereals.

Thornalley, P.J., Babaei-Jadidi, R., Al Ali, H. *et al.* High prevalence of low plasma thiamine concentration in diabetes linked to a marker of vascular disease. *Diabetologia* **50**, 2164–2170 (2007). doi.10.1007/s00125-007-0771-4.

Tryon MS, Stanhope KL, Epel ES, Mason AE, Brown R, Medici V, Havel PJ, Laugero KD. Excessive Sugar Consumption May Be a Difficult Habit to Break: A View From the Brain and Body. J Clin Endocrinol Metab. 2015 Jun;100(6):2239-47. doi: 10.1210/jc.2014-4353.

Tsitouras PD, Gucciardo F, Salbe AD, Heward C, Harman SM. High omega-3 fat intake improves insulin sensitivity and reduces CRP and IL6, but does not affect other endocrine axes in healthy older adults. Horm Metab Res. 2008 Mar;40(3):199-205. doi: 10.1055/s-2008-1046759.

Tsitouras PD, Gucciardo F, Salbe AD, Heward C, Harman SM. High omega-3 fat intake improves insulin sensitivity and reduces CRP and IL6, but does not affect other endocrine axes in healthy older adults. Horm Metab Res. 2008 Mar;40(3):199-205. doi: 10.1055/s-2008-1046759.

Chapter 7: Ultra-processed Foods

Adjibade M, Julia C, Allès B, Touvier M, Lemogne C, Srour B, Hercberg S, Galan P, Assmann KE, Kesse-Guyot E. Prospective association between ultra-processed food consumption and incident depressive symptoms in the French NutriNet-Santé cohort. BMC Med. 2019 Apr 15;17(1):78. doi: 10.1186/s12916-019-1312-y.

Bratanova B, Loughnan S, Klein O, Claassen A, Wood R. Poverty, inequality, and increased consumption of high calorie food: Experimental evidence for a causal link. Appetite. 2016 May 1;100:162-71. doi: 10.1016/j.appet.2016.01.028.

Brown, A. 2020. FAT CHANCE: Boris Johnson says 'I was too fat' as he reveals 'obesity plan'. The *Sun*. Retrieved from: https://www.thesun.co.uk/news/12233916/boris-johnson-fat-obesity/.

Cornwell B, Villamor E, Mora-Plazas M, Marin C, Monteiro CA, Baylin A. Processed and ultra-processed foods are associated with lower-quality nutrient profiles in children from Colombia.PublicHealthNutr.2018Jan;21(1):142-147.doi:10.1017/S1368980017000891.

Department of Health and Social Care. 2020. New obesity strategy unveiled as country urged to lose weight to beat coronavirus (COVID-19) and protect the NHS. Retrieved from: https://www.gov.uk/government/news/new-obesity-strategy-unveiled-as-country-urged-to-lose-weight-to-beat-coronavirus-covid-19-and-protect-the-nhs.

Department of Health and Social Care. 2020. Tackling obesity: empowering adults and children to live healthier lives. Retrieved from: https://www.gov.uk/government/publications/tackling-obesity-government-strategy/tackling-obesity-empowering-adults-and-children-to-live-healthier-lives.

Dimbleby, H. 2021. National Food Strategy. Independent Review.

Filippa Juul, Niyati Parekh, Euridice Martinez-Steele, Carlos Augusto Monteiro, Virginia W Chang, Ultra-processed food consumption among US adults from 2001 to 2018, *The American Journal of Clinical Nutrition*, Volume 115, Issue 1, January 2022, Pages 211–221, https://doi.org/10.1093/ajcn/nqab305.

Finnis, A. 2022. When did Boris Johnson have Covid? How long PM was in hospital and timeline of the Downing Street party row. I News. Retrieved from: https://inews.co.uk/news/boris-johnson-covid-when-have-hospital-how-long-dates-timeline-downing-street-party-row-1393965.

Food Foundation. 2020. Broken Plate 2020: the state of the nation's food system Technical Report.

Food Foundation. 2020. 'Broken Plate 2020: the state of the nation's food system: At a glance'. Retrieved from: https://foodfoundation.org.uk/sites/default/files/2022-07/FF_BP_AT%20A%20GLANCE.pdf.

Gómez-Donoso C, Sánchez-Villegas A, Martínez-González MA, Gea A, Mendonça RD, Lahortiga-Ramos F, Bes-Rastrollo M. Ultra-processed food consumption and the incidence of depression in a Mediterranean cohort: the SUN Project. Eur J Nutr. 2020 Apr;59(3):1093-1103. doi: 10.1007/s00394-019-01970-1.

Google Trends. Retrieved from: https://trends.google.com/trends/explore?date=today%205-y&geo=GB&q=underlying%20health%20condition.

Hague, W. 2022. Obesity U-turn is weak, shallow and immoral. *The Sunday Times*. Retrieved from: https://www.thetimes.co.uk/article/this-obesity-u-turn-shames-our-ministers-pvdfbkp5k.

Hayhoe R, Rechel B, Clark AB, Gummerson C, Smith SJL, Welch AA. Cross-sectional associations of schoolchildren's fruit and vegetable consumption, and meal choices, with their mental well-being: a cross-sectional study. BMJ Nutr Prev Health. 2021 Sep 27;4(2):447-462. doi: 10.1136/bmjnph-2020-000205.

Jacka FN, Cherbuin N, Anstey KJ, Sachdev P, Butterworth P. Western diet is associated with a smaller hippocampus: a longitudinal investigation. BMC Med. 2015 Sep 8;13:215. doi: 10.1186/s12916-015-0461-x.

Lordan R. Dietary supplements and nutraceuticals market growth during the coronavirus pandemic - Implications for consumers and regulatory oversight. PharmaNutrition. 2021 Dec;18:100282. doi: 10.1016/j.phanu.2021.100282.

Louzada ML, Martins AP, Canella DS, Baraldi LG, Levy RB, Claro RM, Moubarac JC, Cannon G, Monteiro CA. Impact of ultra-processed foods on micronutrient content in the Brazilian diet. Rev Saude Publica. 2015;49:45. doi: 10.1590/S0034-8910.2015049006211.

Marrón-Ponce JA, Sánchez-Pimienta TG, Rodríguez-Ramírez S, Batis C, Cediel G. Ultra-processed foods consumption reduces dietary diversity and micronutrient intake in the Mexican population. J Hum Nutr Diet. 2022 Mar 12. doi: 10.1111/jhn.13003.

Mertens E, Colizzi C, Peñalvo JL. Ultra-processed food consumption in adults across Europe. Eur J Nutr. 2022 Apr;61(3):1521-1539. doi: 10.1007/s00394-021-02733-7.

Ministry of Heath of Brazil. 2015. Dietary Guidelines for the Brazilian Population.

Monteiro, C.A., Cannon, G., Levy, R.B., Moubarac, J., Jaime, P.C., Martins, A.P., Canella, D.S., Louzada, M.L., & Parra, D.C. (2016). NOVA. The star shines bright.

Mordor Intelligence. 'Functional Food Market – Growth, Trends, Covid-19 Impact, and Forecasts (2022 – 2027)'. Retrieved from: https://www.mordorintelligence.com/industry-reports/global-functional-food-market.

NIHR School for Public Health Research. 2021. Urgent action needed to reduce harm of ultra-processed foods to British children. Retrieved from: https://sphr.nihr.ac.uk/news-and-events/news/urgent-action-needed-to-reduce-harm-of-ultra-processed-foods-to-british-children/.

Novak D, Štefan L, Prosoli R, Emeljanovas A, Mieziene B, Milanović I, Radisavljević-Janić S. Mediterranean Diet and Its Correlates among Adolescents in Non-Mediterranean European Countries: A Population-Based Study. Nutrients. 2017 Feb 22;9(2):177. doi: 10.3390/nu9020177.

Rauber F, Steele EM, Louzada MLDC, Millett C, Monteiro CA, Levy RB. Ultra-processed food consumption and indicators of obesity in the United Kingdom population (2008-2016). PLoS One. 2020 May 1;15(5):e0232676. doi: 10.1371/journal.pone.0232676.

Roberts, C. 2014. Fruit and vegetable consumption. *Health Survey for England*. Retrieved from: http://healthsurvey.hscic.gov.uk/media/1092/_7-fruit-and-vegetable-consumption_7th-proof.pdf.

Robinsons Orange Squash No Added Sugar 1L.https://www.sainsburys.co.uk/gol-ui/product/robinsons-squash-orange--no-added-sugar-1l.

Schraer, R. 2020. Coronavirus: Smokers quit in highest numbers in a decade. BBC News. Retrieved from: https://www.bbc.co.uk/news/health-53403610.

Shubrook, N. 'The health benefits of oranges'. *BBC Good Food*. Retrieved from: https://www.bbcgoodfood.com/howto/guide/health-benefits-oranges.

Smithers, R. 2018. Fruit and veg used in scheme for English schools 'often inedible'. Retrieved from: https://www.theguardian.com/education/2018/nov/27/fruit-and-veg-used-in-scheme-for-english-schools-often-inedible.

Stevenson RJ, Francis HM, Attuquayefio T, Gupta D, Yeomans MR, Oaten MJ, Davidson T. Hippocampal-dependent appetitive control is impaired by experimental exposure to a Western-style diet. R Soc Open Sci. 2020 Feb 19;7(2):191338. doi: 10.1098/rsos.191338.

The *Guardian*. 2020. 'I shook hands with everybody,' says Boris Johnson weeks before coronavirus diagnosis – video. Retrieved from: https://www.theguardian.com/world/video/2020/mar/27/i-shook-hands-with-everybody-says-boris-johnson-weeks-before-coronavirus-diagnosis-video.

United Stated Department for Agriculture. 2017. The fresh fruit and vegetable programme. https://fns-prod.azureedge.us/sites/default/files/resource-files/FFVPFactSheet.pdf.

Walker, P. 2020. Boris Johnson missed five coronavirus Cobra meetings, Michael Gove says. The *Guardian*. Retrieved from: https://www.theguardian.com/world/2020/apr/19/michael-gove-fails-to-deny-pm-missed-five-coronavirus-cobra-meetings.

Chapter 8: Psychobiotics

Bourassa MW, Alim I, Bultman SJ, Ratan RR. Butyrate, neuroepigenetics and the gut microbiome: Can a high fiber diet improve brain health? Neurosci Lett. 2016 Jun 20;625:56-63. doi: 10.1016/j.neulet.2016.02.009.

Hantsoo L, Jašarević E, Criniti S, McGeehan B, Tanes C, Sammel MD, Elovitz MA, Compher C, Wu G, Epperson CN. Childhood adversity impact on gut microbiota and inflammatory response to stress during pregnancy. Brain Behav Immun. 2019 Jan;75: 240-250. doi: 10.1016/j.bbi.2018.11.005.

Kazemi A, Noorbala AA, Azam K, Eskandari MH, Djafarian K. Effect of probiotic and prebiotic vs placebo on psychological outcomes in patients with major depressive disorder: A randomized clinical trial. Clin Nutr. 2019 Apr;38(2):522-528. doi: 10.1016/j.clnu.2018.04.010.

Köhler O, Petersen L, Mors O, Mortensen PB, Yolken RH, Gasse C, Benros ME. Infections and exposure to anti-infective agents and the risk of severe mental disorders: a nationwide study. Acta Psychiatr Scand. 2017 Feb;135(2):97-105. doi: 10.1111/acps.12671.

Lavebratt C, Yang LL, Giacobini M, Forsell Y, Schalling M, Partonen T, Gissler M. Early exposure to antibiotic drugs and risk for psychiatric disorders: a population-based study. Transl Psychiatry. 2019 Nov 26;9(1):317. doi: 10.1038/s41398-019-0653-9.

Lurie I, Yang YX, Haynes K, Mamtani R, Boursi B. Antibiotic exposure and the risk for depression, anxiety, or psychosis: a nested case-control study. J Clin Psychiatry. 2015 Nov;76(11):1522-8. doi: 10.4088/JCP.15m09961.

Madison AA, Belury MA, Andridge R, Renna ME, Rosie Shrout M, Malarkey WB, Lin J, Epel ES, Kiecolt-Glaser JK. Omega-3 supplementation and stress reactivity of cellular aging biomarkers: an ancillary substudy of a randomized, controlled trial in midlife adults. Mol Psychiatry. 2021 Jul;26(7):3034-3042. doi: 10.1038/s41380-021-01077-2.

McDonald D, Hyde E, Debelius JW, Morton JT, Gonzalez A, Ackermann G, Aksenov AA, Behsaz B, Brennan C, Chen Y, DeRight Goldasich L, Dorrestein PC, Dunn RR, Fahimipour AK, Gaffney J, Gilbert JA, Gogul G, Green JL, Hugenholtz P, Humphrey G, Huttenhower C, Jackson MA, Janssen S, Jeste DV, Jiang L, Kelley ST, Knights D, Kosciolek T, Ladau J, Leach J, Marotz C, Meleshko D, Melnik AV, Metcalf JL, Mohimani H, Montassier E, Navas-Molina J, Nguyen TT, Peddada S, Pevzner P, Pollard KS, Rahnavard G, Robbins-Pianka A, Sangwan N, Shorenstein J, Smarr L, Song SJ, Spector T, Swafford AD, Thackray VG, Thompson LR, Tripathi A, Vázquez-Baeza Y, Vrbanc A, Wischmeyer P, Wolfe E, Zhu Q; American Gut Consortium, Knight R. American Gut: an Open Platform for Citizen Science Microbiome Research. mSystems. 2018 May 15;3(3):e00031-18. doi: 10.1128/mSystems.00031-18.

Müller B, Rasmusson AJ, Just D, Jayarathna S, Moazzami A, Novicic ZK, Cunningham JL. Fecal Short-Chain Fatty Acid Ratios as Related to Gastrointestinal and Depressive Symptoms in Young Adults. Psychosom Med. 2021 Sep 1;83(7):693-699. doi: 10.1097/PSY.0000000000000965.

NHS. 'How to get more fibre into your diet'. Retrieved from https://www.nhs.uk/live-well/eat-well/digestive-health/how-to-get-more-fibre-into-your-diet/on 5 November 2022.

Public Health England. 2020. National Diet and Nutrition Survey Rolling programme Years 9 to 11 (2016/2017 to 2018/2019).

Reemst K, Tims S, Yam KY, Mischke M, Knol J, Brul S, Schipper L, Korosi A. The Role of the Gut Microbiota in the Effects of Early-Life Stress and Dietary Fatty Acids on Later-Life Central and Metabolic Outcomes in Mice. mSystems. 2022 Jun 28;7(3):e0018022. doi: 10.1128/msystems.00180-22.

Schaub, AC., Schneider, E., Vazquez-Castellanos, J.F. *et al*. Clinical, gut microbial and neural effects of a probiotic add-on therapy in depressed patients: a randomized controlled trial. *Transl Psychiatry* **12**, 227 (2022). https://doi.org/10.1038/s41398-022-01977-z.

Shapira, M. 2016. 'Gut Microbiotas and Host Evolution: Scaling Up Symbiosis'. *Trends in Ecology & Evolution*, 31(7), 539–549. doi:10.1016/j.tree.2016.03.006.

Thompson, J.M., K.E. Waldie, C.R. Wall, R. Murphy, E.A. Mitchell; ABC study group. 'Associations between acetaminophen use during pregnancy and ADHD symptoms measured at ages 7 and 11 years'. *PLoS One*. 24 Sep 2014;9(9):e108210. doi: 10.1371/journal.pone.0108210. PMID: 25251831; PMCID: PMC4177119.

Chapter 9: Alcohol

Alcázar A, Pablos F, Martín MA, González AG. Multivariate characterisation of beers according to their mineral content. Talanta. 2002 Apr 22;57(1):45-52. doi: 10.1016/s0039-9140(01)00670-1.

Ammar, A., K. Trabelsi, O. Boukhris, B. Bouaziz, P. Müller, J. Glenn, N.T. Bott, N. Müller, H. Chtourou, T. Driss, A. Hökelmann. 'Effects of Polyphenol-Rich Interventions on Cognition and Brain Health in Healthy Young and Middle-Aged Adults: Systematic Review and Meta-Analysis'. *J Clin Med*. 25 May 2020;9(5):1598. doi: 10.3390/jcm9051598. PMID: 32466148; PMCID: PMC7290428.

Department of Health & Social Care. 2021. Guidance: Fetal alcohol spectrum disorder: health needs assessment. Retrieved from: https://www.gov.uk/government/publications/fetal-alcohol-spectrum-disorder-health-needs-assessment/fetal-alcohol-spectrum-disorder-health-needs-assessment#fn:3.

Fiona McAndrew, Jane Thompson, Lydia Fellows, Alice Large, Mark Speed and Mary J. Renfrew. 2012. Infant Feeding Survey 2010.

Gibson GE, Hirsch JA, Fonzetti P, Jordan BD, Cirio RT, Elder J. Vitamin B1 (thiamine) and dementia. Ann N Y Acad Sci. 2016 Mar;1367(1):21-30. doi: 10.1111/nyas.13031.

Lamport DJ, Pal D, Moutsiana C, Field DT, Williams CM, Spencer JP, Butler LT. 'The effect of flavanol-rich cocoa on cerebral perfusion in healthy older adults during conscious resting state: a placebo controlled, crossover, acute trial'. *Psychopharmacology* (Berl). Sep 2015;232(17):3227-34. doi: 10.1007/s00213-015-3972-4. Epub 2015 Jun 7. PMID: 26047963; PMCID: PMC4534492.

Netmums. 2021. Can you drink Guinness when pregnant? Retrieved from: https://www.netmums.com/pregnancy/can-you-drink-guinness-when-pregnant.

NHS Digital. 2020. Statistics on Alcohol, England 2020. Retrieved from: https://digital.nhs.uk/data-and-information/publications/statistical/statistics-on-alcohol/2020.

NHS Digital. 2020. Statistics on Alcohol, England 2020. Retrieved from: https://digital.nhs.uk/data-and-information/publications/statistical/statistics-on-alcohol/2020/part-1#estimated-alcohol-related-hospital-admissions-narrow-measure.

Nykjaer C, Alwan NA, Greenwood DC, Simpson NA, Hay AW, White KL, Cade JE. Maternal alcohol intake prior to and during pregnancy and risk of adverse birth outcomes: evidence from a British cohort. J Epidemiol Community Health. 2014 Jun;68(6):542-9. doi: 10.1136/jech-2013-202934.

Office for Health Improvement and Disparities. 2021. Official Statistics. Local Alcohol Profiles for England: short statistical commentary, October 2021. Retrieved from: https://www.gov.uk/government/statistics/local-alcohol-profiles-for-england-lape-october-2021-update/local-alcohol-profiles-for-england-short-statistical-commentary-october-2021.

Office for National Statistics. 2018. Adult drinking habits in Great Britain: 2017. Retrieved from: https://www.ons.gov.uk/peoplepopulationandcommunity/health andsocialcare/drugusealcoholandsmoking/bulletins/opinionsandlifestylesur veyadultdrinkinghabitsingreatbritain/2017.

Phan HTT, Samarat K, Takamura Y, Azo-Oussou AF, Nakazono Y, Vestergaard MC. 'Polyphenols Modulate Alzheimer's Amyloid Beta Aggregation in a Structure-Dependent Manner'. *Nutrients*. 31 Mar 2019;11(4):756. doi: 10.3390/nu11040756. PMID: 30935135; PMCID: PMC6521010.

Popova S, Lange S, Probst C, Gmel G, Rehm J. Estimation of national, regional, and global prevalence of alcohol use during pregnancy and fetal alcohol syndrome: a systematic review and meta-analysis. Lancet Glob Health. 2017 Mar;5(3):e290-e299. doi: 10.1016/S2214-109X(17)30021-9.

Ridley NJ, Draper B, Withall A. 'Alcohol-related dementia: an update of the evidence'. *Alzheimers Res Ther*. 25 Jan 2013;5(1):3. doi: 10.1186/alzrt157. PMID: 23347747; PMCID: PMC3580328.

Royal College of Psychiatrists. 2019. Alcohol and depression. Retrieved from: https://www.rcpsych.ac.uk/mental-health/problems-disorders/alcohol-and-depression.

Schneier, F., Foose, T., Hasin, D., Heimberg, R., Liu, S., Grant, B., & Blanco, C. 2010. 'Social anxiety disorder and alcohol use disorder co-morbidity in the National Epidemiologic Survey on Alcohol and Related Conditions'. *Psychological Medicine*, 40(6), 977-988. doi:10.1017/S0033291709991231.

Schwarzinger M, Pollock BG, Hasan OSM, Dufouil C, Rehm J; QalyDays Study Group. Contribution of alcohol use disorders to the burden of dementia in France 2008-13: a nationwide retrospective cohort study. Lancet Public Health. 2018 Mar;3(3):e124-e132. doi: 10.1016/S2468-2667(18)30022-7.

The Royal College of Physicians. 2014. Guinness is good for you? Retrieved from: https://history.rcplondon.ac.uk/blog/guinness-good-you#:~:text=It%20was%20 believed%20to%20be,for%20the%20next%2040%20years.

Walker, P. 2021. Chatting over cheese and wine: anatomy of Downing Street lockdown gathering. The Guardian. Retrieved from: https://www.theguardian.com/politics/ 2021/dec/19/chatting-over-cheese-and-wine-anatomy-downing-street-lockdown-gathering-picture.

World Health Organisation. 2020. Alcohol pricing in the WHO European Region: update report on the evidence and recommended policy actions (2020).

Chapter 10: Food, school exclusion and the cycle of poverty

Andrews, J., Birrell, L., Chapman, C., Teesson, M., Newton, N., Allsop, S., . . . Slade, T. (2022). Evaluating the effectiveness of a universal eHealth school-based prevention programme for depression and anxiety, and the moderating role of friendship network characteristics. *Psychological Medicine*, 1-10. doi:10.1017/S0033291722002033.

BBC News. 2020. Conservative MP quits government job over free school meals. Retrieved from: https://www.bbc.co.uk/news/uk-politics-54642788.

Cardiff University. 'The truth about in-work poverty'. Retrieved from: https://www.cardiff.ac.uk/research/features/the-truth-about-in-work-poverty.

Chefs in School. 2022. Survation Chefs in Schools 2022 Survey. Retrieved from: https://chefsinschools.org.uk/wp-content/uploads/2022/10/Chefs-in-Schools-Summary.pdf.

Chorniy A, Currie J, Sonchak L. 'Does Parental WIC Participation Improve Child Outcomes?' *Am J Health Econ.* 2020 Spring;6(2):169-198. doi: 10.1086/707832.

Clark, D. 2022. Number of people receiving three days' worth of emergency food by Trussell Trust foodbanks in the United Kingdom from 2008/09 to 2021/22. Statista. Retrieved from: https://www.statista.com/statistics/382695/uk-foodbank-users/.

Edmunds D, Wigby S, Perry JC. 'Hangry' *Drosophila*: food deprivation increases male aggression. Anim Behav. 2021 Jul;177:183-190. doi: 10.1016/j.anbehav.2021.05.001.

Gailliot, Matthew. (2013). Hunger and Reduced Self-Control in the Laboratory and across the World: Reducing Hunger as a Self-Control Panacea. Psychology. 04. 59-66. 10.4236/psych.2013.41008.

Galler JR, Bryce CP, Waber DP, Hock RS, Harrison R, Eaglesfield GD, Fitzmaurice G. Infant malnutrition predicts conduct problems in adolescents. Nutr Neurosci. 2012 Jul;15(4):186-92. doi: 10.1179/1476830512Y.0000000012.

Hansen, J. 2020. 322 MPs Voted Against Extending Free School Meal Vouchers to Easter 2021. Eater London. Retrieved from: https://london.eater.com/2020/10/22/21528125/free-school-meals-extension-government-vote-against.

Liu J, Raine A, Venables PH, Mednick SA. 'Malnutrition at age 3 years and external-izing behavior problems at ages 8, 11, and 17 years'. *Am J Psychiatry.* Nov 2004;161(11):2005-13. doi: 10.1176/appi.ajp.161.11.2005. PMID: 15514400; PMCID: PMC1570126.

Jones NR, Conklin AI, Suhrcke M, Monsivais P. The growing price gap between more and less healthy foods: analysis of a novel longitudinal UK dataset. PLoS One. 2014 Oct 8;9(10):e109343. doi: 10.1371/journal.pone.0109343.

Krabbendam L, Bakker E, Hornstra G, van Os J. Relationship between DHA status at birth and child problem behaviour at 7 years of age. Prostaglandins Leukot Essent Fatty Acids. 2007 Jan;76(1):29-34. doi: 10.1016/j.plefa.2006.09.004.

Learmonth, A. 2021. Tories ditch Glasgow candidate who said food bank users are 'far from starving'. The National. Retrieved from: https://www.thenational.scot/news/19013530.tories-suspend-glasgow-pollok-candidate-claimed-food-bank-users-far-starving/.

National Audit Office. 2020. 'Report – Value for money. Investigation into government procurement during the COVID-19 pandemic'. Retrieved from: https://www.nao.org.uk/reports/government-procurement-during-the-covid-19-pandemic/#concluding-remarks.

National Statistics. 2022. Permanent exclusions and suspensions in England. Retrieved from: https://explore-education-statistics.service.gov.uk/find-statistics/permanent-and-fixed-period-exclusions-in-england.

Niccolò Fattorini, Claudia Brunetti, Carolina Baruzzi, Elisabetta Macchi, Maria Chiara Pagliarella, Noemi Pallari, Sandro Lovari, Francesco Ferretti, Being "hangry": food depletion and its cascading effects on social behaviour, *Biological Journal of the Linnean*

Society, Volume 125, Issue 3, November 2018, Pages 640–656, https://doi.org/10.1093/biolinnean/bly119.

Office for National Statistics. 2018. Human capital estimates, UK: 2004 to 2017 https://www.ons.gov.uk/peoplepopulationandcommunity/wellbeing/articles/humancapitalestimates/2004to2017.

Office for National Statistics. 2022. 'Health inequalities. Current patterns and trends in ill health and death by measures of socio-economic status'. Retrieved from: https://www.ons.gov.uk/peoplepopulationandcommunity/healthandsocialcare/healthinequalities.

Oxfam India. 2021. Inequality Report 2021: India's Unequal Healthcare Story Retrieved from: https://www.oxfamindia.org/knowledgehub/workingpaper/inequality-report-2021-indias-unequal-healthcare-story.

Parnham, J.C.; Chang, K.; Rauber, F.; Levy, R.B.; Millett, C.; Laverty, A.A.; von Hinke, S.; Vamos, E.P. 2022. 'The Ultra-Processed Food Content of School Meals and Packed Lunches in the United Kingdom'. *Nutrients* 14, 2961. https://doi.org/10.3390/nu14142961.

Pogrund, D & Calver, T. 2020. Chumocracy first in line as ministers splash Covid cash. The Sunday Times. Retrieved from: https://www.thetimes.co.uk/article/chumocracy-first-in-line-as-ministers-splash-covid-cash-7wb5b8q0w.

Siddiqui F, Salam RA, Lassi ZS, Das JK. The Intertwined Relationship Between Malnutrition and Poverty. Front Public Health. 2020 Aug 28;8:453. doi: 10.3389/fpubh.2020.00453.

Travis, A. 2017. 'Public services face real-terms spending cuts of up to 40% in decade to 2020'. The *Guardian*. Retrieved from: https://www.theguardian.com/uk-news/2017/nov/22/public-services-face-real-terms-spending-cuts-of-up-to-40-in-decade-to-2020.

UK Parliament. 'Plan your event'. Retrieved from: https://www.parliament.uk/visiting/venue-hire/commons/planning/.

Sunter, R. 2022. Expanding free school meals: a cost benefit analysis. Retrieved from: https://urbanhealth.org.uk/insights/reports/expanding-free-school-meals-a-cost-benefit-analysis.

Swami V, Hochstöger S, Kargl E, Stieger S. Hangry in the field: An experience sampling study on the impact of hunger on anger, irritability, and affect. PLoS One. 2022 Jul 6;17(7):e0269629. doi: 10.1371/journal.pone.0269629.

The Health Foundation. 2020. Health Equity in England: The Marmot Review 10 Years On. Retrieved from: https://www.health.org.uk/publications/reports/the-marmot-review-10-years-on.

Williams, M. 2022. Revealed: Lords complain of 'poor wine' and 'too much salmon' in Parliament. Open Democracy. Retrieved from: https://www.opendemocracy.net/en/exclusive-house-of-lords-complaints-food-drink-taxpayer-subsidised/.

World Bank. 2022. Gross domestic product 2021. Retrieved from: https://databank.worldbank.org/data/download/GDP.pdf.

Chapter 11: Crime & Nourishment – The Prison Nutrition Studies

Barth J, Bermetz L, Heim E, Trelle S, Tonia T. The current prevalence of child sexual abuse worldwide: a systematic review and meta-analysis. Int J Public Health. 2013 Jun;58(3):469-83. doi: 10.1007/s00038-012-0426-1.

Bryan K, Freer J, Furlong C. Language and communication difficulties in juvenile offenders. Int J Lang Commun Disord. 2007 Sep-Oct;42(5):505-20. doi: 10.1080/13682820601053977.

Burki T. Crisis in UK prison mental health. Lancet Psychiatry. 2017 Dec;4(12):904. doi: 10.1016/S2215-0366(17)30446-7.

Clark, D. 2021. Average annual overall resource expenditure per prison place in England and Wales from 2015 to 2020. Statista. Retrieved from: https://www.statista.com/statistics/1202172/cost-per-prisoner-england-and-wales/.

Coid, J., Yang, M., Tyrer, P., Roberts, A., & Ullrich, S. (2006). 'Prevalence and correlates of personality disorder in Great Britain'. *British Journal of Psychiatry*, 188(5), 423-431. doi:10.1192/bjp.188.5.423.

Conservatives. 2019. Conservative Party Manifesto 2019. https://www.conservatives.com/our-plan/conservative-party-manifesto-2019.

Devlin, E. 2020. Bidfood parent back in profit ahead of Covid-19 outbreak. The Grocer. Retrieved from: https://www.thegrocer.co.uk/results/bidfood-parent-back-in-profit-ahead-of-covid-19-outbreak/646805.article.

Fazel S, Wolf A. A Systematic Review of Criminal Recidivism Rates Worldwide: Current Difficulties and Recommendations for Best Practice. PLoS One. 2015 Jun 18;10(6):e0130390. doi: 10.1371/journal.pone.0130390.

Firth J, Carney R, Stubbs B, Teasdale SB, Vancampfort D, Ward PB, Berk M, Sarris J. Nutritional Deficiencies and Clinical Correlates in First-Episode Psychosis: A Systematic Review and Meta-analysis. Schizophr Bull. 2018 Oct 17;44(6):1275-1292. doi: 10.1093/schbul/sbx162.

Food Foundation. 2020. Broken Plate 2020: the state of the nation's food system Technical Report.

Gesch, C. B., Hammond, S., Hampson, S., Eves, A., & Crowder, M. (2002). Influence of supplementary vitamins, minerals and essential fatty acids on the antisocial behaviour of young adult prisoners: Randomised, placebo-controlled trial. *British Journal of Psychiatry*, 181(1), 22-28. doi:10.1192/bjp.181.1.22.

HM Government. 2021. UK's greenest and most innovative prison unveiled. Retrieved from: https://www.gov.uk/government/news/uk-s-greenest-and-most-innovative-prison-unveiled.

HM Inspectorate of Prisons. 2016. Life in prison: Food - A findings paper by HM Inspectorate of Prisons. https://www.justiceinspectorates.gov.uk/hmiprisons/wp-content/uploads/sites/4/2016/09/Life-in-prison-Food-Web-2016.pdf.

HM Prison & Probation Service. 2022. Safety in Custody Statistics, England and Wales: Deaths in Prison Custody to June 2022 Assaults and Self-harm to March 2022. Ministry of Justice.

Hongerwinter Onderzoek. https://www.hongerwinter.nl/onderzoek/?lang=en.

House of Commons Committee of Public Accounts. 2017. Mental health in prisons. Eighth Report of Session 2017–19.

Hurley, B. 2021. 'Adverse Childhood Events More Common Among Adults in Prison'. Interrogating Justice. https://interrogatingjustice.org/ending-mass-incarceration/adverse-childhood-events-more-common-among-adults-in-prison/.

Inside Times. 2022. Jump in self-harm rates at women's prisons. Retrieved from: https://insidetime.org/jump-in-self-harm-rates-at-womens-prisons/.

Institute for Government. 2019. Prisons. Retrieved from: https://www.institutefor-government.org.uk/publication/performance-tracker-2019/prisons.

Kim Williams, Vea Papadopoulou and Natalie Booth. 2012. Prisoners' childhood and family backgrounds Results from the Surveying Prisoner Crime Reduction (SPCR) longitudinal cohort study of prisoners.

Lumey LH, Stein AD, Kahn HS, van der Pal-de Bruin KM, Blauw GJ, Zybert PA, Susser ES. 'Cohort profile: the Dutch Hunger Winter families study'. *Int J Epidemiol*. Dec 2007;36(6):1196-204. doi: 10.1093/ije/dym126. Epub 2007 Jun 25. PMID: 17591638.

McKie RM, Sternin S, Kilimnik CD, Levere DD, Humphreys TP, Reesor A, Reissing ED. Nonconsensual Sexual Experience Histories of Incarcerated Men: A Mixed Methods Approach. Int J Offender Ther Comp Criminol. 2021 Dec 19:306624X211065584. doi: 10.1177/0306624X211065584.

Mental Health Foundation. 2022. Diet and Mental Health. Retrieved from: https://www.mentalhealth.org.uk/sites/default/files/food-for-thought-mental-health-nutrition-briefing-march-2017.pdf.

Mental Health Foundation. 2022. 'The most common mental health problems: statistics'. Retrieved from: https://www.mentalhealth.org.uk/explore-mental-health/mental-health-statistics/most-common-mental-health-problems-statistics.

Meyer BJ, Byrne MK, Collier C, Parletta N, Crawford D, Winberg PC, Webster D, Chapman K, Thomas G, Dally J, Batterham M, Farquhar I, Martin AM, Grant L. Baseline omega-3 index correlates with aggressive and attention deficit disorder behaviours in adult prisoners. PLoS One. 2015 Mar 20;10(3):e0120220. doi: 10.1371/journal.pone.0120220.

Meyer BJ, Byrne MK, Cortie CH, Parletta N, Jones A, Eckermann S, Butler T, Greenberg D, Batterham M, Fernandez F, Schofield PW, Winberg PC, Bowles K, Dally J, Martin AM, Grant L. The effect of omega-3 long chain polyunsaturated fatty acids on aggressive behaviour in adult male prisoners: a structured study protocol for a multi-centre, double-blind, randomised placebo-controlled trial and translation into policy and practice. Trials. 2021 May 2;22(1):318. doi: 10.1186/s13063-021-05252-2.

Ministry of Justice. 2012. 'Prisoners' childhood and family backgrounds Results from the Surveying Prisoner Crime Reduction (SPCR) longitudinal cohort study of prisoners'. Retrieved from: https://assets.publishing.service.gov.uk/government/uploads/system/uploads/attachment_data/file/278837/prisoners-childhood-family-backgrounds.pdf.

Ministry of Justice. 2019. Criminal Justice Statistics quarterly: December 2019. Retrieved from: https://www.gov.uk/government/statistics/criminal-justice-system-statistics-quarterly-december-2019/criminal-justice-statistics-quarterly-december-2019-html.

Ministry of Justice. National Statistics. 2021. Prison population projections: 2021 to 2026. Retrieved from: https://www.gov.uk/government/statistics/prison-population-projections-2021-to-2026.

Ministry of Justice. 2022. 'Transparency data. Prison population figures: 2022'. Population bulletin: weekly 26 August 2022. Retrieved from: https://www.gov.uk/government/publications/prison-population-figures-2022.

National Audit Office. 2006. Report – Value for Money. Serving Time: Prisoner Diet and Exercise. Retrieved from: https://www.nao.org.uk/report/serving-time-prisoner-diet-and-exercise/.

National Audit Office. 2017. Report – Value for money: Mental health in prisons. Retrieved from: https://www.nao.org.uk/reports/mental-health-in-prisons/.

National Literacy Trust. 2017. Adult literacy: Information on adult literacy in the UK and our Books Unlocked programme. Retrieved from: https://literacytrust.org.uk/parents-and-families/adult-literacy/.

NSPCC. 2021. Statistics briefing: child sexual abuse. Retrieved from: https://learning.nspcc.org.uk/media/1710/statistics-briefing-child-sexual-abuse.pdf.

Painter, R., Osmond, C., Gluckman, P., Hanson, M., Phillips, D. and Roseboom, T. 2008. 'Transgenerational effects of prenatal exposure to the Dutch famine on neonatal adiposity and health in later life'. *BJOG: An International Journal of Obstetrics & Gynaecology*, 115: 1243-1249. https://doi.org/10.1111/j.1471-0528.2008.01822.x.

PrisonUK. 2014. Prison UK: An Insider's View. Retrieved from: https://prisonuk.blogspot.com/2014/09/prison-food-glorious-food.html.

Public Health England. 2016. 'Psychosis Data Report. Describing variation in numbers of people with psychosis and their access to care in England'. Retrieved from: https://assets.publishing.service.gov.uk/government/uploads/system/uploads/attachment_data/file/774680/Psychosis_data_report.pdf.

Raine, A., Leung, CC., Singh, M. *et al*. Omega-3 supplementation in young offenders: a randomized, stratified, double-blind, placebo-controlled, parallel-group trial. *J Exp Criminol* **16**, 389–405 (2020). https://doi.org/10.1007/s11292-019-09394-x.

Savage, M. 2021. 'Deep crisis' in British prisons as use of force against inmates doubles. The Guardian. Retrieved from: https://www.theguardian.com/society/2021/jan/03/deep-crisis-british-prisons-use-force-inmates-overcrowding.

Schoenthaler, S., S. Amos, W. Doraz, M-A. Kelly, G. Muedeking, J. Wakefield Jr (1997) 'The Effect of Randomized Vitamin-Mineral Supplementation on Violent and Non-violent Antisocial Behavior Among Incarcerated Juveniles, *Journal of Nutritional & Environmental Medicine*, 7:4, 343-352, DOI: 10.1080/13590849762475.

UK Government. 1999. The Prison Rules 1999. Retrieved from: https://www.legislation.gov.uk/uksi/1999/728/article/24.

Veenendaal, M, Painter, R, de Rooij, S, Bossuyt, P, van der Post, J, Gluckman, P, Hanson, M, Roseboom, T. 'Transgenerational effects of prenatal exposure to the 1944–45 Dutch famine'. *BJOG*. 2013; 120: 548– 554.

Walker T, Shaw J, Gibb J, Turpin C, Reid C, Gutridge K, Abel K. Lessons Learnt From the Narratives of Women Who Self-Harm in Prison. Crisis. 2021 Jul;42(4):255-262. doi: 10.1027/0227-5910/a000714.

World Prison Brief. 2022. Highest to Lowest - Prison Population Total. Retrieved from: https://www.prisonstudies.org/highest-to-lowest/prison-population-total?field_region_taxonomy_tid=14.

Zaalberg A, Nijman H, Bulten E, Stroosma L, van der Staak C. Effects of nutritional supplements on aggression, rule-breaking, and psychopathology among young adult prisoners. Aggress Behav. 2010 Mar-Apr;36(2):117-26. doi: 10.1002/ab.20335.

Chapter 12: Nutrition and mood

Adjibade M, Lemogne C, Touvier M, Hercberg S, Galan P, Assmann KE, Julia C, Kesse-Guyot E. The Inflammatory Potential of the Diet is Directly Associated with Incident Depressive Symptoms Among French Adults. J Nutr. 2019 Jul 1;149(7): 1198-1207. doi: 10.1093/jn/nxz045.

Bayes J, Schloss J, Sibbritt D. The effect of a Mediterranean diet on the symptoms of depression in young males (the "AMMEND: A Mediterranean Diet in MEN with

Depression" study): a randomized controlled trial. Am J Clin Nutr. 2022 Aug 4;116(2): 572-580. doi: 10.1093/ajcn/nqac106.

Brown, C.C., Raio, C.M. & Neta, M. Cortisol responses enhance negative valence perception for ambiguous facial expressions. *Sci Rep* 7, 15107 (2017). https://doi.org/10.1038/s41598-017-14846-3.

Bushman BJ, Dewall CN, Pond RS Jr, Hanus MD. Low glucose relates to greater aggression in married couples. Proc Natl Acad Sci U S A. 2014 Apr 29;111(17):6254-7. doi: 10.1073/pnas.1400619111.

Moufidath Adjibade, Cédric Lemogne, Mathilde Touvier, Serge Hercberg, Pilar Galan, Karen E Assmann, Chantal Julia, Emmanuelle Kesse-Guyot, The Inflammatory Potential of the Diet is Directly Associated with Incident Depressive Symptoms Among French Adults, *The Journal of Nutrition*, Volume 149, Issue 7, July 2019, Pages 1198–1207, https://doi.org/10.1093/jn/nxz045.

Parletta N, Zarnowiecki D, Cho J, Wilson A, Bogomolova S, Villani A, Itsiopoulos C, Niyonsenga T, Blunden S, Meyer B, Segal L, Baune BT, O'Dea K. A Mediterranean-style dietary intervention supplemented with fish oil improves diet quality and mental health in people with depression: A randomized controlled trial (HELFIMED). Nutr Neurosci. 2019 Jul;22(7):474-487. doi: 10.1080/1028415X.2017.1411320.

Rucklidge JJ, Andridge R, Gorman B, Blampied N, Gordon H, Boggis A. Shaken but unstirred? Effects of micronutrients on stress and trauma after an earthquake: RCT evidence comparing formulas and doses. Hum Psychopharmacol. 2012 Sep;27(5):440-54. doi: 10.1002/hup.2246.

Rucklidge JJ, Eggleston MJF, Johnstone JM, Darling K, Frampton CM. Vitamin-mineral treatment improves aggression and emotional regulation in children with ADHD: a fully blinded, randomized, placebo-controlled trial. J Child Psychol Psychiatry. 2018 Mar;59(3):232-246. doi: 10.1111/jcpp.12817.

Rucklidge JJ, Frampton CM, Gorman B, Boggis A. Vitamin-mineral treatment of attention-deficit hyperactivity disorder in adults: double-blind randomised placebo-controlled trial. Br J Psychiatry. 2014;204:306-15. doi: 10.1192/bjp.bp.113.132126.

Sarris J, Murphy J, Mischoulon D, Papakostas GI, Fava M, Berk M, Ng CH. Adjunctive Nutraceuticals for Depression: A Systematic Review and Meta-Analyses. Am J Psychiatry. 2016 Jun 1;173(6):575-87. doi: 10.1176/appi.ajp.2016.15091228.

Verhaak PFM, de Beurs D, Spreeuwenberg P. 'What proportion of initially prescribed antidepressants is still being prescribed chronically after 5 years in general practice? A longitudinal cohort analysis'. BMJ Open, 2019;9:e024051. doi: 10.1136/bmjopen-2018-024051.

Chapter 13: Neurodegeneration

Allen, LH. 'How common is vitamin B-12 deficiency?' *The American Journal of Clinical Nutrition*, Volume 89, Issue 2, February 2009, Pages 693S–696S, https://doi.org/10.3945/ajcn.2008.26947A.

Amen DG, Harris WS, Kidd PM, Meysami S, Raji CA. Quantitative Erythrocyte Omega-3 EPA Plus DHA Levels are Related to Higher Regional Cerebral Blood Flow on Brain SPECT. J Alzheimers Dis. 2017;58(4):1189-1199. doi: 10.3233/JAD-170281.

Barbagallo M, Veronese N, Dominguez LJ. Magnesium in Aging, Health and Diseases. Nutrients. 2021 Jan 30;13(2):463. doi: 10.3390/nu13020463.

Borsini A, Stangl D, Jeffries AR, Pariante CM, Thuret S. The role of omega-3 fatty acids in preventing glucocorticoid-induced reduction in human hippocampal neurogenesis and increase in apoptosis. Transl Psychiatry. 2020 Jul 7;10(1):219. doi: 10.1038/s41398-020-00908-0.

Carter, Janet. (2022). Prevalence of all cause young onset dementia and time lived with dementia: analysis of primary care health records. Journal of Dementia Care. 30.

de Baaij JH, Hoenderop JG, Bindels RJ. Magnesium in man: implications for health and disease. Physiol Rev. 2015 Jan;95(1):1-46. doi: 10.1152/physrev.00012.2014.

Cazzola R, Della Porta M, Manoni M, Iotti S, Pinotti L, Maier JA. 'Going to the roots of reduced magnesium dietary intake: A tradeoff between climate changes and sources'. *Heliyon*. 3 Nov 2020;6(11):e05390. doi: 10.1016/j.heliyon.2020.e05390. PMID: 33204877; PMCID: PMC7649274.

Department of Health and Social Care. 2022. Policy paper. Our plan for patients. Retrieved from: https://www.gov.uk/government/publi cations/our-plan-for-patients/ our-plan-for-patients#care.

DiNicolantonio JJ, O'Keefe JH. The Importance of Marine Omega-3s for Brain Development and the Prevention and Treatment of Behavior, Mood, and Other Brain Disorders. Nutrients. 2020 Aug 4;12(8):2333. doi: 10.3390/nu12082333.

Freund-Levi Y, Eriksdotter-Jönhagen M, Cederholm T, Basun H, Faxén-Irving G, Garlind A, Vedin I, Vessby B, Wahlund LO, Palmblad J. Omega-3 fatty acid treatment in 174 patients with mild to moderate Alzheimer disease: OmegAD study: a randomized double-blind trial. Arch Neurol. 2006 Oct;63(10):1402-8. doi: 10.1001/archneur.63.10.1402.

Graham, L., Harder, J., Soto, I. *et al.* Chronic consumption of a western diet induces robust glial activation in aging mice and in a mouse model of Alzheimer's disease. *Sci Rep* 6, 21568 (2016). https://doi.org/10.1038/srep21568.

Gudala K, Bansal D, Schifano F, Bhansali A. Diabetes mellitus and risk of dementia: A meta-analysis of prospective observational studies. J Diabetes Invcstig. 2013 Nov 27;4(6):640-50. doi: 10.1111/jdi.12087.

Harris WS, Tintle NL, Imamura F, Qian F, Korat AVA, Marklund M, Djoussé L, Bassett JK, Carmichael PH, Chen YY, Hirakawa Y, Küpers LK, Laguzzi F, Lankinen M, Murphy RA, Samieri C, Senn MK, Shi P, Virtanen JK, Brouwer IA, Chien KL, Eiriksdottir G, Forouhi NG, Geleijnse JM, Giles GG, Gudnason V, Helmer C, Hodge A, Jackson R, Khaw KT, Laakso M, Lai H, Laurin D, Leander K, Lindsay J, Micha R, Mursu J, Ninomiya T, Post W, Psaty BM, Risérus U, Robinson JG, Shadyab AH, Snetselaar L, Sala-Vila A, Sun Y, Steffen LM, Tsai MY, Wareham NJ, Wood AC, Wu JHY, Hu F, Sun Q, Siscovick DS, Lemaitre RN, Mozaffarian D; Fatty Acids and Outcomes Research Consortium (FORCE). Blood n-3 fatty acid levels and total and cause-specific mortality from 17 prospective studies. Nat Commun. 2021 Apr 22;12(1):2329. doi: 10.1038/s41467-021-22370-2.

Jernerén F, Elshorbagy AK, Oulhaj A, Smith SM, Refsum H, Smith AD. 'Brain atrophy in cognitively impaired elderly: the importance of long-chain ω-3 fatty acids and B vitamin status in a randomized controlled trial'. *Am J Clin Nutr*. Jul 2015;102(1):215-21. doi: 10.3945/ajcn.114.103283. Epub 2015 Apr 15. PMID: 25877495.

Luengo-Fernandez R, Leal J, Gray AM. UK research expenditure on dementia, heart disease, stroke and cancer: are levels of spending related to disease burden? Eur J Neurol. 2012 Jan;19(1):149-54. doi: 10.1111/j.1468-1331.2011.03500.x.

Matsui T, Kihira M, Kobayashi H. 'Experimental studies of skull fracture in the temporal region' (author's transl). No Shinkei Geka. Feb 1975;3(2):123-9. Japanese. PMID: 1238919.

Morris MC, Tangney CC, Wang Y, Sacks FM, Bennett DA, Aggarwal NT. MIND diet associated with reduced incidence of Alzheimer's disease. Alzheimers Dement. 2015 Sep;11(9):1007-14. doi: 10.1016/j.jalz.2014.11.009.

Ngandu T, Lehtisalo J, Solomon A, Levälahti E, Ahtiluoto S, Antikainen R, Bäckman L, Hänninen T, Jula A, Laatikainen T, Lindström J, Mangialasche F, Paajanen T, Pajala S, Peltonen M, Rauramaa R, Stigsdotter-Neely A, Strandberg T, Tuomilehto J, Soininen H, Kivipelto M. A 2 year multidomain intervention of diet, exercise, cognitive training, and vascular risk monitoring versus control to prevent cognitive decline in at-risk elderly people (FINGER): a randomised controlled trial. Lancet. 2015 Jun 6;385(9984): 2255-63. doi: 10.1016/S0140-6736(15)60461-5.

Pottala JV, Yaffe K, Robinson JG, Espeland MA, Wallace R, Harris WS. Higher RBC EPA + DHA corresponds with larger total brain and hippocampal volumes: WHIMS-MRI study. Neurology. 2014 Feb 4;82(5):435-42. doi: 10.1212/WNL. 0000000000000080.

Prasad S, Sajja RK, Naik P, Cucullo L. Diabetes Mellitus and Blood-Brain Barrier Dysfunction: An Overview. J Pharmacovigil. 2014 Jun;2(2):125. doi: 10.4172/ 2329-6887.1000125.

Public Health England. 2020. Official Statistics. NDNS: results from years 9 to 11 (combined) – statistical summary. Retrieved from: https://www.gov.uk/government/statistics/ndns-results-from-years-9-to-11-2016-to-2017-and-2018-to-2019/ndns-results-from-years-9-to-11-combined-statistical-summary.

Sala-Vila A, Satizabal CL, Tintle N, Melo van Lent D, Vasan RS, Beiser AS, Seshadri S, Harris WS. 'Red Blood Cell DHA Is Inversely Associated with Risk of Incident Alzheimer's Disease and All-Cause Dementia: Framingham Offspring Study'. Nutrients. 9 Jun 2022;14(12):2408. doi: 10.3390/nu14122408. PMID: 35745137; PMCID: PMC9228504.

Tan ZS, Harris WS, Beiser AS, Au R, Himali JJ, Debette S, Pikula A, Decarli C, Wolf PA, Vasan RS, Robins SJ, Seshadri S. Red blood cell ω-3 fatty acid levels and markers of accelerated brain aging. Neurology. 2012 Feb 28;78(9):658-64. doi: 10.1212/ WNL.0b013e318249f6a9.

The London School of Economics and Political Science. 2019. Dementia care costs to nearly treble in next two decades. Retrieved from: https://www.lse.ac.uk/News/Latest-news-from-LSE/2019/K-November-2019/Dementia-care.

Toffa DH, Magnerou MA, Kassab A, Hassane Djibo F, Sow AD. Can magnesium reduce central neurodegeneration in Alzheimer's disease? Basic evidences and research needs. Neurochem Int. 2019 Jun;126:195-202. doi: 10.1016/j.neuint.2019.03.014.

Veronese N, Zurlo A, Solmi M, Luchini C, Trevisan C, Bano G, Manzato E, Sergi G, Rylander R. Magnesium Status in Alzheimer's Disease: A Systematic Review. Am J Alzheimers Dis Other Demen. 2016 May;31(3):208-13. doi: 10.1177/ 1533317515602674.

Woltil, H., van Beusekom, C., Schaafsma, M. et al. Red Blood Cell Docosahexaenoic Acid (Rbc Dha) Status 6 Weeks After Birth Is Related To Early Brain Growth in Low-Birth-Weight Infants 252. Pediatr Res 40, 557 (1996). https://doi.org/10.1203/ 00006450-199609000-00275.

Xue M, Xu W, Ou YN, Cao XP, Tan MS, Tan L, Yu JT. Diabetes mellitus and risks of cognitive impairment and dementia: A systematic review and meta-analysis of 144 prospective studies. Ageing Res Rev. 2019 Nov;55:100944. doi: 10.1016/j. arr.2019.100944.

Chapter 14: Veganism and brain health

Gibson RA, Muhlhausler B, Makrides M. Conversion of linoleic acid and alpha-linolenic acid to long-chain polyunsaturated fatty acids (LCPUFAs), with a focus on pregnancy, lactation and the first 2 years of life. Matern Child Nutr. 2011 Apr;7 Suppl 2(Suppl 2):17-26. doi: 10.1111/j.1740-8709.2011.00299.x.

Hovinen T, Korkalo L, Freese R, Skaffari E, Isohanni P, Niemi M, Nevalainen J, Gylling H, Zamboni N, Erkkola M, Suomalainen A. Vegan diet in young children remodels metabolism and challenges the statuses of essential nutrients. EMBO Mol Med. 2021 Feb 5;13(2):e13492. doi: 10.15252/emmm.202013492.

Iguacel I, Huybrechts I, Moreno LA, Michels N. Vegetarianism and veganism compared with mental health and cognitive outcomes: a systematic review and meta-analysis. Nutr Rev. 2021 Mar 9;79(4):361-381. doi: 10.1093/nutrit/nuaa030.

Kocaoglu C, Akin F, Caksen H, Böke SB, Arslan S, Aygün S. 'Cerebral atrophy in a vitamin B12-deficient infant of a vegetarian mother'. *J Health Popul Nutr.* Jun 2014;32(2):367-71. PMID: 25076673; PMCID: PMC4216972.

Lövblad K, Ramelli G, Remonda L, Nirkko AC, Ozdoba C, Schroth G. Retardation of myelination due to dietary vitamin B12 deficiency: cranial MRI findings. Pediatr Radiol. 1997 Feb;27(2):155-8. doi: 10.1007/s002470050090.

Neufingerl N, Eilander A. 'Nutrient Intake and Status in Adults Consuming Plant-Based Diets Compared to Meat-Eaters: A Systematic Review'. Nutrients. Dec 23 2021;14(1):29. doi: 10.3390/nu14010029.

The Vegan Society. 2022. Worldwide growth of veganism. Retrieved from: https://www.vegansociety.com/news/media/statistics/worldwide.

The Vegan Society. Vitamin B12. Retrieved from: https://www.vegansociety.com/resources/nutrition-and-health/nutrients/vitamin-b12.

Tong TYN, Appleby PN, Bradbury KE, Perez-Cornago A, Travis RC, Clarke R, Key TJ. Risks of ischaemic heart disease and stroke in meat eaters, fish eaters, and vegetarians over 18 years of follow-up: results from the prospective EPIC-Oxford study. BMJ. 2019 Sep 4;366:l4897. doi: 10.1136/bmj.l4897.

Vegan Health. B12 Deficiency Cases in Vegan Infants and Toddlers. Retrieved from: https://veganhealth.org/vitamin-b12/b12-deficiency-cases-in-vegan-infants-and-toddlers/.

Viva. 2022. 'Statistics about veganism'. Retrieved from: https://viva.org.uk/lifestyle/statistics-about-veganism/.

Whelan J, Fritsche K. Linoleic acid. Adv Nutr. 2013 May 1;4(3):311-2. doi: 10.3945/an.113.003772.

Wunsch, N-G. 2020. Share of adults who follow a vegan diet in Great Britain in 2019, by gender and age group. Statista. Retrieved from: https://www.statista.com/statistics/1062343/adults-following-vegan-diet-in-great-britain-by-gender-and-age/.

Chapter 15: The Psychology of Food Choice

Bruce AS, Holsen LM, Chambers RJ, Martin LE, Brooks WM, Zarcone JR, Butler MG, Savage CR. Obese children show hyperactivation to food pictures in brain networks linked to motivation, reward and cognitive control. Int J Obes (Lond). 2010 Oct;34(10):1494-500. doi: 10.1038/ijo.2010.84.

Hall KD, Ayuketah A, Brychta R, Cai H, Cassimatis T, Chen KY, Chung ST, Costa E, Courville A, Darcey V, Fletcher LA, Forde CG, Gharib AM, Guo J, Howard R, Joseph PV, McGehee S, Ouwerkerk R, Raisinger K, Rozga I, Stagliano M, Walter M, Walter PJ, Yang S, Zhou M. Ultra-Processed Diets Cause Excess Calorie Intake and Weight Gain: An Inpatient Randomized Controlled Trial of Ad Libitum Food Intake. Cell Metab. 2019 Jul 2;30(1):67-77.e3. doi: 10.1016/j.cmet.2019.05.008. Epub 2019 May 16. Erratum in: Cell Metab. 2019 Jul 2;30(1):226. Erratum in: Cell Metab. 2020 Oct 6;32(4):690.

Statista. 2020. Most common types of stress experienced in the United Kingdom (UK) in 2020* Retrieved from: https://www.statista.com/statistics/1134359/common-types-of-stress-in-the-uk/.

Teo PS, Lim AJ, Goh AT, R J, Choy JYM, McCrickerd K, Forde CG. Texture-based differences in eating rate influence energy intake for minimally processed and ultra-processed meals. Am J Clin Nutr. 2022 Jul 6;116(1):244-254. doi: 10.1093/ajcn/nqac068.

Yau A, Berger N, Law C, Cornelsen L, Greener R, Adams J, Boyland EJ, Burgoine T, de Vocht F, Egan M, Er V, Lake AA, Lock K, Mytton O, Petticrew M, Thompson C, White M, Cummins S. Changes in household food and drink purchases following restrictions on the advertisement of high fat, salt, and sugar products across the Transport for London network: A controlled interrupted time series analysis. PLoS Med. 2022 Feb 17;19(2):e1003915. doi: 10.1371/journal.pmed.1003915.

Chapter 16: The Persistent Myth of the Nanny State

Ambrose, T. 2022. 'Sunak faces backlash over delay to junk food pre-watershed ads ban'. *The Guardian*. Retrieved from: https://www.theguardian.com/business/2022/dec/08/sunak-faces-backlash-over-delay-to-junk-food-pre-watershed-ads-ban.

Barton, C. 2017. Research Briefing: Home ownership and renting: demographics. UK Parliament. Retrieved from: https://commonslibrary.parliament.uk/research-briefings/cbp-7706/.

BBC News. 2018. 'Food waste crackdown 'to help serve up 250m meals'. Retrieved from: https://www.bbc.co.uk/news/uk-politics-45705843.

Bone, J., Sloan, M., Brown, H., Behrendt, Hannah., Goozee, Z., Harper, H., Tankelevitch, Lev. & Farrington, J. 2021. Changing Minds about Changing Behaviours: Obesity in focus. Nesta. Available from: https://media.nesta.org.uk/documents/changing-minds_about_changing_behaviours_Xi5X9RC.pdf.

Cabinet Office. 2012. Government's nudge unit goes global. Retrieved from: https://www.gov.uk/government/news/governments-nudge-unit-goes-global.

Centers for Disease Control and Prevention. 2021. Tobacco and cancer. Retrieved from: https://www.cdc.gov/cancer/tobacco/index.htm.

Connolly, G. 2022. Carrier bag tax raises £37m for NI environmental projects. BBC News. Retrieved from: https://www.bbc.co.uk/news/uk-northern-ireland-60946194

Davidson, P. 2022. Clip of Rishi Sunak boasting he took money from 'deprived areas' to help wealthy towns resurfaces. Daily Record. Retrieved from: https://www.dailyrecord.co.uk/news/politics/clip-rishi-sunak-boasting-took-28313445.

Davies, R. 2020. UK tobacco sales fell faster after plain packaging rules came into force. The Guardian. Retrieved from: https://www.theguardian.com/society/2020/jul/13/uk-tobacco-sales-fell-faster-after-plain-packaging-rules-came-into-force-cigarettes.

Department for Environment, Food & Rural Affairs and The Rt Hon Michael Gove MPUK Government. 2018. 'Action to reduce food waste announced'. Retrieved from: https://www.gov.uk/government/news/action-to-reduce-food-waste-announced.

Department for Environment, Food & Rural Affairs. 2021. Policy paper. Carrier bags: why there's a charge. Retrieved from: https://www.gov.uk/govern ment/publica-tions/single-use-plastic-carrier-bags-why-were-introducing-the-charge/carrier-bags-why-theres-a-5p-charge.

European Commission. 2014. Public Health. Product Regulation. Tobacco Products Directive (2014/40/EU). Retrieved from: https://health.ec.europa.eu/tobacco/product-regulation_en.

Francis-Devine, B., Irvine, S. & Gorb, A. 2022. Food Banks in the UK. UK Parlia ment. House of Commons Library. Retrieved from: https://commonslibrary.parliament.uk/research-briefings/cbp-8585/.

GBD 2017 Diet Collaborators. Health effects of dietary risks in 195 countries, 1990-2017: a systematic analysis for the Global Burden of Disease Study 2017. Lancet. 2019 May 11;393(10184):1958-1972. doi: 10.1016/S0140-6736(19)30041-8. Epub 2019 Apr 4. Erratum in: Lancet. 2021 Jun 26;397(10293):2466.

HM Government. 2011. No health without mental health A cross-government mental health outcomes strategy for people of all ages.

HM Revenue & Customs. 2022. 'Official Statistics Soft Drinks Industry Levy: Statistics commentary 2022'. Retrieved from: https://www.gov.uk/government/statistics/soft-drinks-industry-levy-statistics/soft-drinks-industry-levy-statistics-commentary-2021.

Institute for Government. 2020. "Nudge Unit". Retrieved from: https://www.insti-tuteforgovernment.org.uk/explainers/nudge-unit.

Medicines and Healthcare products Regulatory Agency. 2012. Best practice guidance on the sale of medicines for pain relief.

Neville, S & Pickard, J. 2016. UK tax on sugary drinks is 'nannying' and 'impractical'. The Financial Times. Retrieved from: https://www.ft.com/content/5b41e47a-ec53-11e5-bb79-2303682345c8.

Office for National Statistics. 2018. Contracts that do not guarantee a minimum num-ber of hours: April 2018. Retrieved from: https://www.ons.gov.uk/employ mentandlabourmarket/peopleinwork/earningsandworkinghours/articles/contract-sthatdonotguaranteeaminimumnumberofhours/april2018.

Office for National Statistics. 2022. 'Dataset(s): Young adults living with their parents'. Retrieved from: https://www.ons.gov.uk/peoplepopulationandcommunity/births-deathsandmarriages/families/datasets/youngadultslivingwiththeirparents/current.

Slawson, N. 2017. Second-home ownership up 30% since 2000, research finds. The Guardian. Retrieved from: https://www.theguardian.com/money/2017/aug/19/second-home-ownership-up-30-since-2000-research-finds.

Sleight, S. 2022. Jeremy Hunt's Autumn Statement: 10 Things To Expect. *Huffington Post*. Retrieved from: https://www.huffingtonpost.co.uk/entry/jeremy-hunt-autumn-statement-what-to-expect_uk_6359431de4b051268c5b2faf.

Smyth, C. 2022. NHS doesn't need cash, says Steve Barclay. *The Times*. Retrieved from: https://www.thetimes.co.uk/article/nhs-doesnt-need-cash-says-steve-barclay-999nrh5cz?

Stevens, J., Warren, J. & Wilcock, D. 2022. Liz Truss vows to halt Nanny State ban on BOGOF deals: Tory leadership candidate pledges no new taxes on food that's high in fat, salt or sugar if she wins battle to be next PM. *Mail Online*. Retrieved from. https://

www.dailymail.co.uk/news/article-11069973/Liz-Truss-vows-halt-Nanny-State-ban-buy-one-one-free-deals-stop-taxes-unhealthy-food.html.

The Equality Trust. 2019. The Scale of Economic Inequality in the UK. Retrieved from: https://equalitytrust.org.uk/scale-economic-inequality-uk.

The Health Foundation. Policy Navigator. 'Report on the sanitary conditions of the labouring population of Great Britain'. Retrieved from: https://navigator.health.org.uk/theme/report-sanitary-conditions-labouring-population-great-britain.

The London School of Economics and Political Science. 2022. Mental health problems cost UK economy at least £118 billion a year - new research. Retrieved from: https://www.lse.ac.uk/News/Latest-news-from-LSE/2022/c-Mar-22/Mental-health-problems-cost-UK-economy-at-least-118-billion-a-year-new-research.

Tommy's. 'Planning for Pregnancy Tool'. Retrieved from: https://www.tommys.org/pregnancy-information/planning-pregnancy/planning-for-pregnancy-tool December 2022.

Truss, E. 2019. On the Nanny State – FREER. Conservatives. Retrieved from: https://www.elizabethtruss.com/news/nanny-state-freer.

UK Parliament. 1977. Hansard. Road Traffic (Seat Belts) Bill Hl Volume 382: debated on Tuesday 26 April 1977. Retrieved from: https://navigator.health.org.uk/theme/report-sanitary-conditions-labouring-population-great-britain.

UK Parliament. 2015. 'The Standardised Packaging of Tobacco Products Regulations 2015'. Retrieved from: https://www.legislation.gov.uk/uksi/2015/829/contents/made.

UK Preconception Partnership. 2022. Retrieved from: https://www.ukpreconception-partnership.co.uk/ December 2022.

UK supermarkets sign government pledge to help halve food waste. Retrieved from. https://www.gov.uk/government/news/uk-supermarkets-sign-government-pledge-to-help-halve-food-waste.

United Nations. 'Do you know all 17 SDGs?' Retrieved from: https://sdgs.un.org/goals.

van Rookhuijzen M, de Vet E. 'Nudging healthy eating in Dutch sports canteens: a multi-method case study'. *Public Health Nutr*. 2021 Feb;24(2):327-337. doi: 10.1017/S1368980020002013.

Which? 2018. '35 years of car seat belts – how have they made a difference?' Retrieved from:https://www.which.co.uk/news/article/35-years-of-car-seat-belts-how-have-they-made-a-difference-agvvP5p97wYc.

World Food Summit. 1996. Rome Declaration. on World Food Security. Retrieved from: https://www.fao.org/3/w3613e/w3613e00.htm.

World Health Organisation. 2021. Targets and Indicators List. Retrieved from: https://cdn.who.int/media/docs/default-source/ncds/ncd-surveillance/who-gmf-targets-and-indicators-list.pdf?sfvrsn=4dcf2a55_1&download=true.

Appendix

Finnish Food Authority. 2021. Adults. Retrieved from: https://www.ruokavirasto.fi/en/themes/healthy-diet/nutrition-and-food-recommendations/adults/.

INDEX

Note: page numbers in **bold** refer to diagrams, page numbers in *italics* refer to information contained in tables.

Conservatives 121, 125, 159–60, 167, 171, 240–3, 254
cortical thickness 63, 69
corticosteroids 156
cortisol 53, 96–7, 136, 156, 190–1
'cost of living crisis' 120, 122, 124–5, 158, 161, 243–4
Covid-19 pandemic 8–9, 75, 94, 116–20, 124, 159–60, 232, 242, 254–5
cranial volume 32, *32*
cravings 49, 97, 192–3, 232
Crawford, Michael 50
cretinism 42
crime *see* prisons
cultural norms 49
cultural shifts 246–7
Currie, Edwina 242
cytokines 30, 97–8, 101, 132, 135, 138, 201

dairy alternatives 219
death 9, 94, 212
decision architects 237, 255–6
decision-making 11, 236–7, 240
dementia 9, 197–212, 245
  and alcohol consumption 146–8, 151
  and the blood-brain barrier 200–3
  and diabetes 93–4, 102, 201–6
  frontotemporal *199*
  and hypothyroidism 44
  interventions 206–11
  and iodine insufficiency 44
  with Lewy bodies *198*
  prevention 102
  risk factors for 146–7, 199
  and sugar 102
  types of 93, *198–9*
  and ultra-processed foods 111, 113, 208
  vascular 93, *198*, 202
  young-onset (YOD) 147–8, 202–3
  see also Alzheimer's disease
demonic possession 15–16
Denmark 61, 136
deoxyribonucleic acid (DNA) 178, 209
Department of Agriculture, Fresh Fruit and Vegetable Program (FFVP) 114
Department of Health 123, 142
Department of Health and Social Care 100
depression 7, 11, 15, 20, 180, 185–93, 245
  and alcohol consumption 149
  and antibiotics 135–6

  carers and 211
  causes of 18–19, 187
  and childhood experience 137–8
  children and 154
  diagnosis 17–18
  disease burden of 185
  and gestational diabetes 95
  and homocysteine 72
  inflammation hypothesis of 187–8, 201
  mild/moderate 19
  and premature birth 52
  and prisons 174
  and probiotics 134–5
  risk of developing 15
  serotonin hypothesis of 19, 185, 187
  severe 19, 186
  and stress 188–91
  and sugar 101, 102
  symptoms 17–18
  treatment-resistant 8, 185
  and ultra-processed foods 112, 185, 187
  and veganism/vegetarianism 220
deprivation 57–8, 98, 114–15, 123, 125, 163–4
Descartes, René 17, 21
developmental disorders 36, 255
diabetes 91–5, 97, 102, 104, 167, 254
  and dementia 93–4, 102, 201–6
  gestational 47, 94–5
  and omega-3 fatty acids 98–9
  type 1 91, 94
  type 2 91, 93–6, 99, 201–2, 209–10, 258
  'type 3' 203–6
Diagnostic and Statistical Manual of Mental Disorders (DSM) 17–18
Dickens, Charles 118
dietary inflammatory index (DII) 188
dietary recommendations 257–8
Dimbleby, Henry 115
discrimination 164
distress 8, 11, 16, 180, 253
docosahexaenoic acid (DHA) 3, 27–34, 30, 45, 47, 49–72, 107, 137, 215
  biomagnification 50
  and breast milk 56–7, 67
  and children 154
  and choline 75–9
  deficiency 29, 50
  and dementia 204–7
  functions 50–66
  and IQ 59–66